Drinkable Healing Herbal Infusions

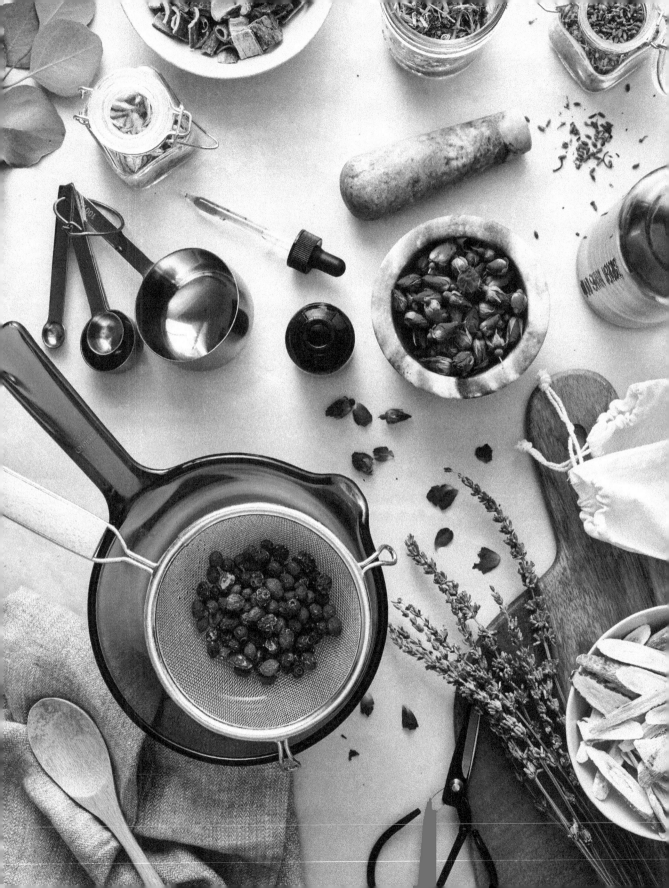

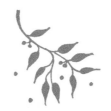

DRINKABLE HEALING
Herbal Infusions

100 BEVERAGES TO SOOTHE YOUR AILMENTS AND BOOST YOUR IMMUNITY

Brighid Doherty

ROCKRIDGE
PRESS

First Rockridge Press trade paperback edition 2022

Rockridge Press and the Rockridge Press logo are trademarks or registered trademarks of Callisto Media Inc. and/or its affiliates in the United States and other countries and may not be used without written permission.

For general information on our other products and services, please contact our Customer Care Department within the United States at (866) 744-2665, or outside the United States at (510) 253-0500.

Paperback ISBN: 978-1-63878-480-7 | ebook ISBN: 978-1-63878-660-3

Manufactured in the United States of America

Interior and Cover Designer: Jenny Paredes
Art Producer: Sara Feinstein
Editor: Adrian Potts
Production Editor: Ashley Polikoff
Production Manager: Riley Hoffman

Cover photography © 2022 Marija Vidal. Interior photography © Alicia Cho, p. ii, 8, 32, 39, 40; Lucia Loiso, p. x, xii; Hélène Dujardin, p. 2; Annie Martin, p. 42; Biz Jones, p. 58; Evi Abeler, p. 74, 166. All other photography used under license from Shutterstock.com.

10 9 8 7 6 5 4 3 2 1 0

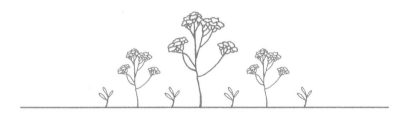

This book is dedicated to my daughter, Isla Rose.
May you carry the wisdom of herbalism forward
to future generations.

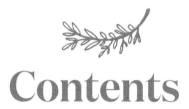

Contents

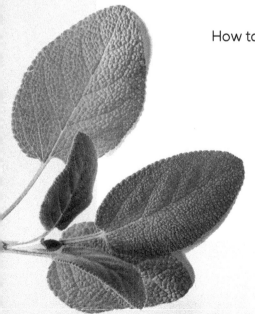

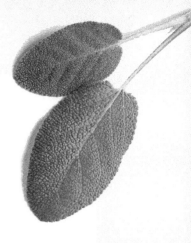

PART II:
Healing Herbal Infusions

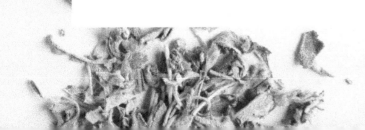

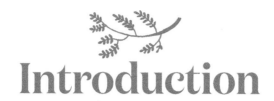

Introduction

My passion for herbalism started in my mother's garden. As a kid, I loved to get down on my hands and knees to examine intricate flowers and inhale their fragrance. Those moments began my lifelong fascination with plants that sustains my love of herbalism today.

Herbalism is the art and science of working with herbs as food and medicine. When I was a freshman in college in the mid '90s, I became aware that herbs had a role as medicine, but I didn't realize herbalism could be a professional calling. I remember hearing a friend announcing she was going to study herbalism. A spark ignited within me. "Herbalism is a *thing*!?" I thought. "I want to be an herbalist!"

Since then, I have had a growing passion for improving heatlh by understanding and working with plants. I have learned from multiple mentors with vastly different approaches to herbalism, which gives me a broad spectrum of understanding to build from in my herbal pursuits.

Since I began my formal education in herbalism, I have managed a natural pharmacy, interned on a medicinal herb farm, offered private health consultations, taught workshops, and led medicinal plant walks. In 2018, I founded the Solidago School of Herbalism and now host *The Healthy Herb Podcast*, both of which are designed to inform and inspire the home herbalist. I teach how to simply incorporate herbs into everyday living. I make an array of home remedies for myself, my family, and friends from plants that I forage, grow, and purchase.

Incorporating herbs into everyday living has brought me joy, health, and an appreciation of the plant world. I love being able to step outside my door and relate to the common plants that grow all around me. Plants that are typically considered noxious weeds and sprayed with poisons are often health-promoting plants. When we shift our understanding of these plants and realize the many gifts of health they offer, we improve the health of ourselves, our communities, and the land to which we belong.

Herbal medicine has been used for thousands of years. It is a major element of alternative medicine and is useful in preventing and treating a number of common ailments. However, in the modern era, in industrialized pockets of the world, many have lost their relationship with healing plants. Now, there is an ever-growing desire to reconnect with these lost relations. The ancient and necessary role of the home herbalist is being reclaimed. Nature's pharmacy is extensive, filled with herbs that possess powerful medicinal properties. With guidance and knowledge, everyone can use herbs to strengthen their health and build resiliency.

In this book, you will begin the journey of the home herbalist via one of the simplest and most enjoyable means: creating safe, nourishing, and enjoyable herbal beverages. The 100 recipes provided here use some of the world's most common and effective herbs in all manner of beverages and liquids, including teas, tonics, syrups, and more.

Although it was once difficult to buy medicinal herbs, they are now much easier to find at well-stocked pharmacies, on the shelves of big-box stores, and in the aisles of health-food stores. They can often be purchased at an affordable cost. Even if you don't have easy access to some herbs, popular online distributors offer all the ingredients you need. Some herbs may even be already hiding inside your spice cabinet! There is also the option to grow and harvest fresh herbs yourself.

This book offers an entrance to a rich and rewarding relationship between you and the healing power of plants. After reading this book and working with the recipes, you, the home herbalist, will be informed, inspired, and empowered in your own health care.

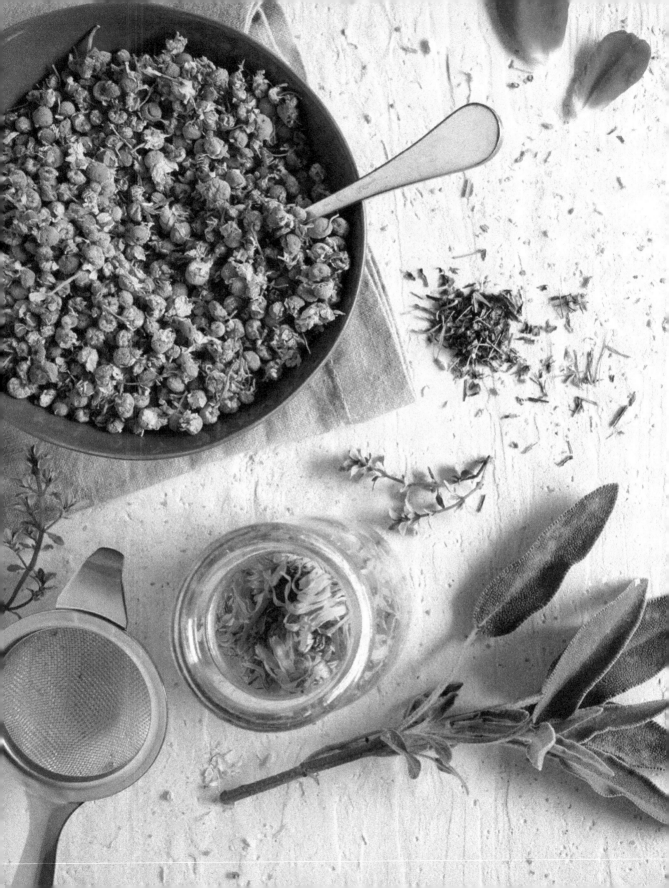

How to Use this Book

This book is divided into two parts. Part 1 will give you the basic information you need to get started with making delicious healing herbal beverages. It contains easy reference guides that will support you on your journey. These guides include helpful kitchen tools, base ingredients for your infusions, the top 15 herbs we will work with, how to acquire the herbs, and the types of drinkable infusions you will be making.

Part 2 contains recipes for herbal beverages organized by the body systems they benefit most. You will notice that the top 15 herbs we talk about in part 1 are found in recipes for multiple body systems. Herbs are complex and varied in their actions. Most herbs enhance many different aspects of our health through the support of multiple body systems.

Herbal medicine is people's medicine. It is simple, safe, and effective, especially when we use herbs in liquid infusions. Even in their simplicity, drinkable herbal infusions can have complex healing effects throughout the body. Still, in cases of pregnancy, severe allergies, and sensitivities, or if you are taking a variety of prescription medications, it is wise to use caution when trying new herbs. Start with small amounts, and see how they make you feel. The herbs in this book are generally safe, food-like herbs, especially when consumed as liquid infused remedies. It is not safe to take herbs in capsule and tablet form, and it is not recommended to ever do so.

It is important to note, also, that these remedies are designed to build health and nutrition and are not intended to replace any medical treatment you may already be receiving. You should still consult with a medical professional if you are concerned about any serious ailments or illnesses.

As you progress through this book, let your intuition, wisdom, and taste buds guide you. Start with the recipes that appeal to you the most, and take it from there. Through this process, you will become more aware of your body, your health, and the herbs that are your best allies.

Are you ready to be a home herbalist for yourself and your loved ones? Let's dig in!

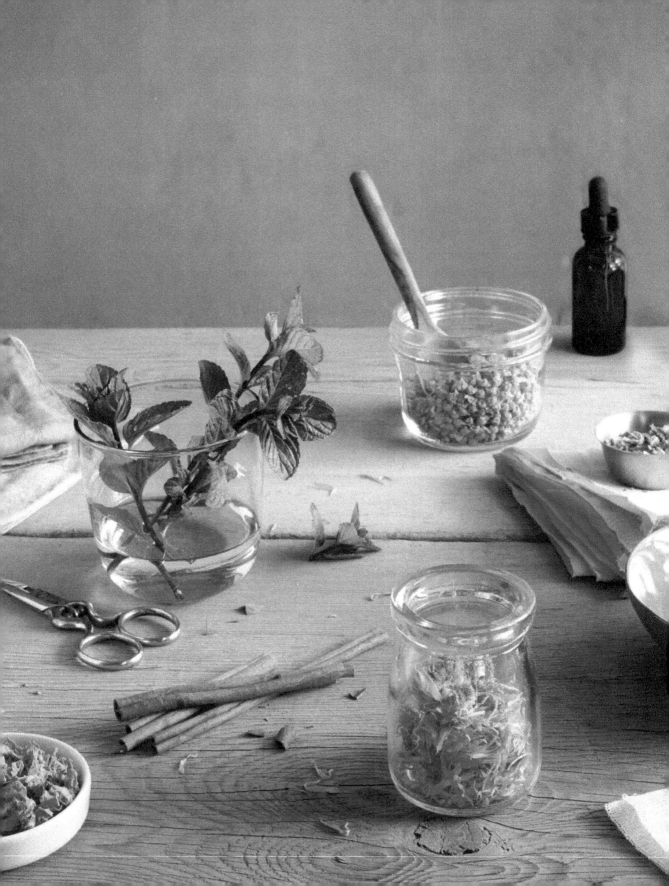

PART I

The Basics of Herbal Infusions

Although herbalism is a vast field of study, the chapters ahead will help you start small and dig deeper as you go. Learning about herbs is like getting to know new friends. Begin by getting to know a few herbs on an individual basis. Taste, smell, and feel how you react to each herb. If the herb grows near you, learn to identify it. Have fun on this journey of exploration; it will be a joyous experience to learn more about yourself and the plants.

This part of the book will provide you with all the information you need to get started. In chapter 1, you will learn the basics of herbalism as a practice and the benefits of home-infused herbal drinks. In chapter 2, you will be introduced to all the tools, ingredients, and herbs you'll need. Chapter 3 will give you more information about the many types of drinkable infusions, along with tips on how to store, label, and dispense your remedies.

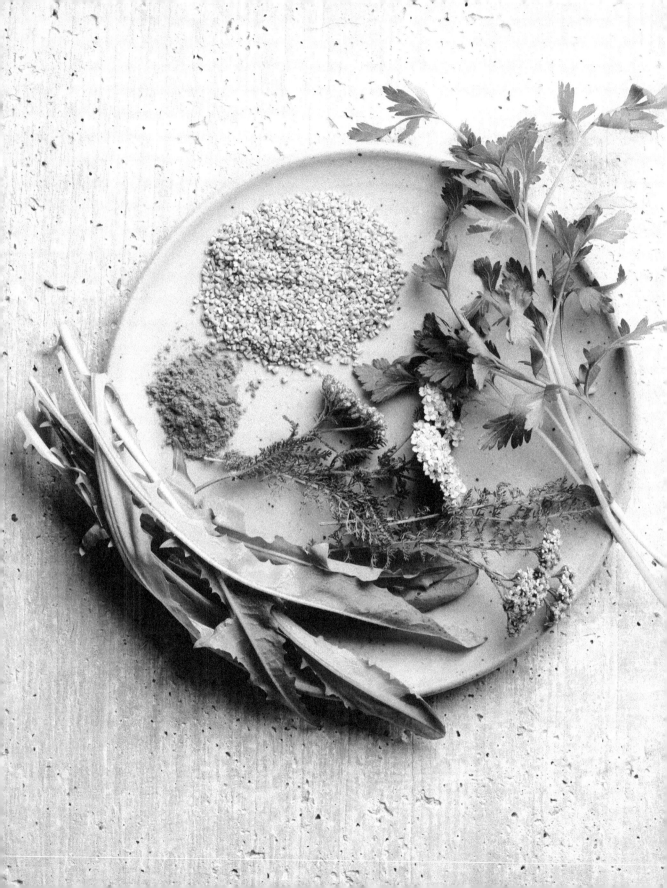

CHAPTER 1

Healing with Herbal Drinks

Herbalism is a tradition of healing that embraces the abilities of plants to improve our health. We improve our mental, physical, and emotional health by adding herbs to our daily life. They increase nutrition, fight infections, improve organ functioning, calm the nerves, and increase resiliency to stress.

Traditionally, herbalism has been the main way humans cared for their health. Historically and in many regions of the world today, caregivers of the household, elders, and midwives use home remedies made from the plants that grow around them to support the health of their families and communities. One of the most time-honored means of consuming these remedies has been by brewing drinks and other liquid herbal preparations.

In modern cultures, we are remembering that herbal medicine is people's medicine. It is a form of health care that we take into our own hands, reclaiming our independence and empowerment in our health.

Holistic Herbal Health

The tradition of herbalism has broad-reaching benefits to our health and well-being. Herbs nourish and optimize our physical functioning with vitamins, minerals, and other important plant constituents. Herbs improve our mental and emotional health.

As we connect with herbs directly in the natural world, their beauty and grace calm and ground our central nervous system. When we sip on a warm cup of sweet, aromatic herbal tea, our mind and nervous system are supported by the simple act of self-care and by the actual plant nutrients that lie within.

Holistic Medicine

Holistic medicine is an approach to health care that supports and nourishes the whole person. It aims to improve well-being by acknowledging and supporting the body, mind, and spirit. Modern medical practice compartmentalizes the body, measuring and attempting to fix individual body systems with pharmaceutical drugs. Herbalism, aligned with a holistic approach, works with plant-based remedies to support all aspects of a person's health and well-being by nourishing their individual wholeness.

Herbs are loaded with minerals and vitamins in forms that our bodies can use for optimum functioning. They also contain secondary metabolites. These are chemicals that the plants do not use for primary functions but that are often used to protect the plants from diseases and pests. They are also used for communication with one another and with other organisms in their ecosystem. Examples of secondary metabolites are the volatile oils that the plants emit as aromas, communicating to insects to either stay away or to come and pollinate. Secondary metabolites also include antioxidants such as bioflavonoids that provide the plants with colors for their flowers and fruits and protect them from the sun and oxidation.

The minerals and vitamins of wild plants offer us nutrition that is important for our physical functions and organ health. The secondary metabolites of plants can protect us from diseases and pathogens, affect our brain and nervous system functions, and protect us from oxidative stress and damage, similarly to how they protect the plants.

Unlike herbal remedies, modern drugs and supplements isolate specific constituents from plants or synthesize similar chemicals in laboratories. This allows people to take specific quantities at a standard dose on a regulated schedule. These drugs tend to have a specific direction of action and, often, side effects that can sometimes harm or challenge the health of the body.

By comparison, when we work with herbs in their whole state to make herbal remedies, we capture the complexity and variation of the plant in that moment. Not only do we include the chemistry of the plant in a complex web of nutrients and secondary metabolites, but also we include the spirit of the plant and the terroir of its environment.

Herbalism as Traditional Medicine

Herbalism has existed since the dawn of humanity. Plants have always provided necessities for human life, including food, fuel, fiber, shelter, spiritual connection, and medicine.

We have coevolved with wild plants through history. Herbs have long been incorporated into spiritual and cultural practices around the world. Even today, they are burned as incense, used to decorate altars, and worshipped as embodiments of nature deities.

Archaeological sites reveal how plants were used in burials, mummification, medicine, and food in different regions. There are ancient human and Neanderthal skulls that have residues of medicinal herbs in their teeth, including a 50,000-year-old Neanderthal tooth with residues of yarrow and chamomile, found in the El Sidrón cave in Spain.

There are various ancient herbal texts from around the world that remain today, including the Egyptian Ebers papyrus (3,500 years old), ancient Indian Ayurveda texts (3,000 years old), and traditional Chinese medicine texts (2,000 years old).

In the first few centuries of the Common Era, alchemists began to separate plant constituents, and so began the journey away from whole-plant medicine toward drug therapy.

However, despite modern drug therapies, herbalism did not disappear, nor did common medicinal weeds. Many in the West are now rediscovering the benefits of these plants for our health and healing. We are seeing the return of the home herbalist and the clinical herbalist in society today.

Benefits of Home-Infused Herbal Drinks

There is a wide range of benefits to incorporating homemade herbal drinks into your daily life. They offer nourishment and healing. They are simple to make, easy to take, cost effective, and safe. Most importantly, you gain empowerment and independence by having the ability to care for your health in simple, delicious, and effective ways. Learning how to make healing herbal drinks is truly life changing!

NATURAL NUTRIENTS: Herbal infusions extract the minerals and vitamins from plants into a drink that we can easily absorb and use the nutrition from. Wild plants and herbs offer a plenitude of vitamins and minerals in natural forms that our bodies can easily assimilate. In fact, once herbs are processed into supplements, powdered, and put into capsules or turned into standardized extracts, they are at their least effective and can come with unwanted side effects.

EASY HYDRATION DURING THE DAY: Herbal drinks are simple to make and easy to consume, especially when they taste delicious. What's more, they can be carried in a thermos, travel mug, or water bottle and sipped throughout a busy day to help keep you hydrated and nourished. They can replace any beverage that may have a negative impact on your health if consumed in excess, such as soda, coffee, or energy drinks. Herbal drinks can also be a great alternative to hydrating your body with water. In fact, when we drink too much pure water, we end up losing minerals from our body due to excessive urination, which in turn messes with the body's electrolyte balance. Drinking nourishing herbal infusions delivers more nutrients to your body to maintain this balance.

LOW COST: Healing herbal drinks made at home are one of the least expensive forms of medicine. Herbs can be purchased at inexpensive rates in bulk from large distributors or in small amounts from your local herb shop. They can also be harvested from your garden or the wild for the cost of your time and effort. On the other hand, herbal supplements, over-the-counter drugs, and prescription medications are often much higher in cost.

No matter your reason for wanting to explore the world of natural remedies, you will be grateful that you are taking the time to learn about these herbs and how to make healing drinks with them. You will know how to increase your nutrition and your health with simple, safe, inexpensive, and effective home-made herbal drinks. You will be able to show your friends and family that making fun and tasty herbal beverages is a delightful way to take health and healing into your own hands.

WILL I ENJOY THESE DRINKS?

Rest assured, you will absolutely enjoy these drinks! Herbs add layers of complex flavors to any beverage. Some healing herbs are bitter or have especially strong flavors, but they can be combined with other, tastier herbs or natural sweeteners to complement their flavor. The more herbal beverages you drink, the more refined your palate will become and the more you will enjoy the variety of flavor herbs offer.

The benefit of making homemade beverages is that you can adjust them to meet your specific taste requirements. The recipes in this book include tips on how to make them taste good to a variety of palates. These healing herbal beverages are easy to make, tasty to drink, and beneficial to your well-being, so you will enjoy incorporating them into your life.

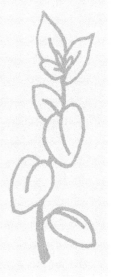

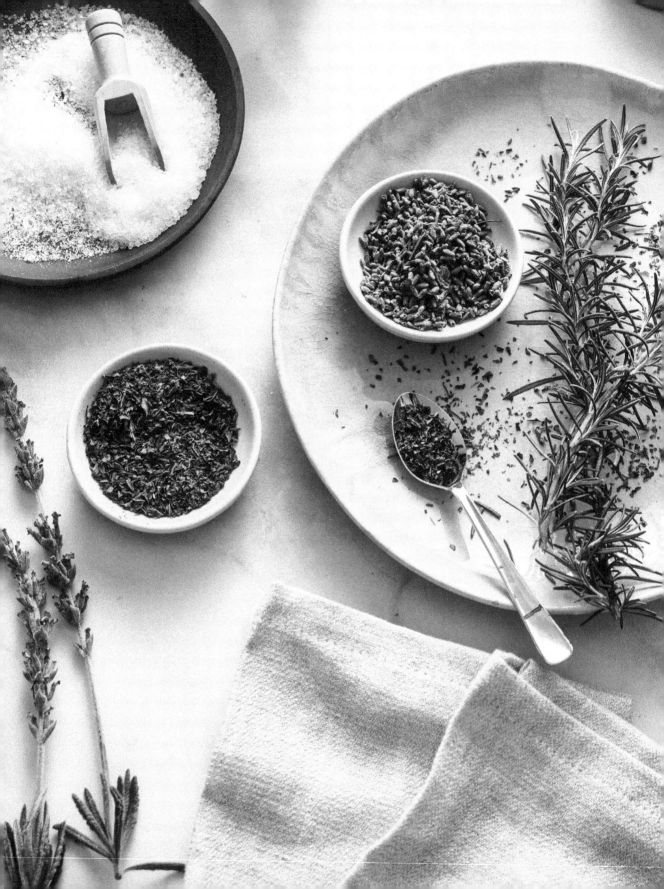

CHAPTER 2

Turning Your Kitchen into an Apothecary

Soon you will be brewing healthy herbal drinks in your own kitchen, but before you get started, you will need some basic tools, pantry staples, and herbs. Having these on hand will help you create any healing herbal beverage whenever you want one. The following is a short list of what to keep in your kitchen. You will likely have many of these already, and what you don't have can be purchased easily at your local variety store or through online retailers.

Tools

Although essential for making healing herbal drinks, none of these kitchen tools is difficult to find or expensive to buy, and you will use them time and time again.

KETTLE: A pot with a lid and spout used for heating and pouring water. An electric kettle works well, too.

COOKING POT: You will need a soup pot or saucepot that holds at least 4 cups of water. A nonmetal—either Pyrex or enamel-lined—pot is used in some recipes for heating vinegar.

TEAPOT: To make many of the recipes, you will need a teapot that holds 4 cups of water. The pots sometimes come with their own strainer, though you can use one without. You can also use a press pot, if you wish.

TEA STRAINER: A sieve tea strainer is used to separate the herb from the tea once it has steeped.

MASON JARS: These jars are used to infuse and store a variety of herbal preparations. Keep a selection of different sizes on hand, including 32-ounce and 16-ounce jars. Metal lids are fine for most recipes; however, to make vinegar infusions, you will need food-safe plastic lids (for 16-ounce mason jars) because vinegar causes metal to rust.

BOSTON ROUND AMBER BOTTLES: These bottles are for storing herbal mixtures such as tinctures and bitters. You will need 8-ounce and 4-ounce bottles. They provide UV protection for light-sensitive products and allow for easy dispensing. It's helpful to have regular caps as well as dropper caps for dispensing. (See page 37 for further notes about dispensing.)

CERAMIC DRIP COFFEE FILTER: Sometimes called a (ceramic) pour-over coffee filter, this tool is used to funnel and strain many infusions in the book.

CLOTH FOR STRAINING: You will need a cloth to line the ceramic drip coffee filter in order to strain infusions. You can use a washable and reusable square piece of cloth made of any natural fiber that has a loose weave. Look for "flour sack" tea towels (usually made from cotton) cut into squares; they work well and are easy to find. Cheesecloth doubled up can also be used but sometimes has too loose a weave and is not reusable.

KITCHEN SCALE: This is used to weigh your herbs. For the recipes in this book, the scale must measure in ounces.

MEASURING SPOONS AND CUPS: Herbs, menstruums (solvent liquids), and remedies are often measured by the teaspoon, tablespoon, or cup. Having 2- and 4-cup liquid measuring cups with a pouring lip is also helpful.

LABELS AND PERMANENT MARKER: You will need labels for preparations such as tinctures, which are stored over longer periods of time, so that you can remember the contents of your bottles. (You may think you'll remember what's in them, but you won't!) You can buy high-quality labels or even use blank address label stickers or masking tape and write on them with a permanent marker.

FUNNEL SET: A variety of different-size small metal funnels will help you transfer freshly strained preparations into bottles without spillage or dripping. A funnel that fits into the neck of a mason jar and has a wide mouth makes it easy to put herbs and even water into the jar when making infusions using 1 ounce of herb.

UNBLEACHED WAX PAPER OR PARCHMENT PAPER: This is sometimes used as a barrier between vinegar infusions and metal lids to prevent the vinegar from rusting the lid.

ELECTRIC BLENDER: This is used for making herb-infused smoothies.

Ingredients

The list of essential nonherb pantry items to make healing herbal drinks is short, and you likely have many of them already. Whatever you don't have can be found at your local grocery and liquor stores.

HONEY: Honey extracts medicine from herbs and is a sweetener. It is used in syrups, elixirs, shrubs, and oxymels.

100-PROOF VODKA: Alcohol is the base of tinctures in this book. One-hundred-proof alcohol is 50 percent alcohol and 50 percent water. It is preferred over 80-proof, which is 40 percent alcohol and 60 percent water. Vodka is preferred because it does not have a flavor of its own and is easily found in 100-proof strength.

APPLE CIDER VINEGAR: This is the vinegar most often used for infusing herbs, though any vinegar other than white vinegar will do.

BUBBLY WATER: This adds fizz to herbal drinks, turning them into sodas or mocktails.

Measuring Your Herbs

Making herbal remedies can be as simple and fun as cooking a healthy meal. As in regular cookbooks, in the recipes in this book, you will see measurements for how much of an herb to use in the infusions.

Keep in mind that herbal medicine is often more of an art than an exact science. Oftentimes, the exact measurement of an herb is not crucial to the effectiveness of the preparations. In these instances, I have used teaspoon, tablespoon, and cup measurements. You can adjust these herb dosages to create delicious and healing remedies that are best suited to your liking and needs.

However, in certain recipes, measuring herbs with a kitchen scale is more important in order to gain the optimum benefit from their nutrients. I have provided these measurements by the ounce. This ensures that you use enough plant material to make an effective preparation. Even with that said, it's important to remember that herbs contain natural variation based on when they were harvested and where they were grown. Due to this natural variation, it is not always possible to create a remedy that is the same every time, which is okay.

Knowing the Right Dosage

Just as when measuring your herbs, knowing the best dosage for your body can take a bit of trial and error. You will find general dosage guidelines listed with each herb description in this chapter and with certain recipes in this book.

For most people, all the herbs in the book are safe in a range of doses, so you can explore what feels right for your body. You can start with the recommended dose, and if you need to, work your way up to a stronger remedy. Safety precautions are included for herbs that may carry risk for people with certain conditions or taking certain medications.

If you are generally sensitive and have strong reactions to foods and drugs, then start with small doses. A small dose could mean a few drops of tincture, a taste of syrup, or a sip of tea. Or you could start by using half of the amount of herbs recommended in the recipes. Be in touch with your body, and see how you feel as you work your way up to a dose that works well for you.

Keep in mind that you should give the herbs time to work. It may take a few days, a few weeks, or even a few months before you notice changes in your health.

The Fantastic 15

The most important part of the healing herbal drinks is, of course, the herbs. The following are profiles of 15 standout herbs that you will find in many recipes in this book. You don't have to stock up on every one of these herbs to start, but it can be good to have them in your home apothecary if you wish to make a range of recipes from this book.

These herbs have been chosen because they are easy to access or harvest on your own and offer a range of health-supporting qualities.

On top of this, they are generally palatable, easy to work with, and enjoyable to consume.

In this section, you will gain an understanding of the broad-reaching benefits that each herb has to offer, which preparations are best suited for them, and any specific considerations with drinking them. (Definitions of unfamiliar terms can be found in the Glossary on page 167.)

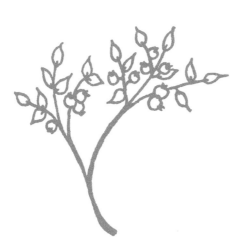

Astragalus

Astragalus membranaceus

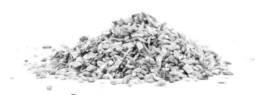

Medicinal part used: root

Properties: adaptogen, antibacterial, antioxidant, antiviral, digestive tonic, heart tonic, immune tonic, kidney tonic, liver tonic, lung tonic, nutritive, restorative

Uses: Astragalus root is best known as a nourishing adaptogen that supports immune function and modulates full-body health. Adaptogen herbs are nontoxic, nonspecific in action, and normalize body functions. Astragalus is an herb to drink when you feel depleted or stressed or are recovering from debility and illness. It improves cardiac blood flow; protects the liver and kidneys; strengthens tendons, bones, and muscles; and enhances physical endurance. Astragalus is helpful for people who have chronic fatigue and fibromyalgia.

Common preparations: decoction, nourishing infusion, food, soup broth, tincture

Common dosage: You can drink up to 1 quart of an astragalus herbal infusion divided throughout the day. You can take 1 dropperful of astragalus tincture 3 times per day or as needed.

TIP: Astragalus root can be purchased in slices that are shaped like a tongue depressor. These can be added to soup stocks, gravies, and rice during cooking to impart medicinal qualities to the food; remove the herb before eating.

Safety considerations: Astragalus membranaceus *is a safe, food-like herb. There are other species of astragalus that are not safe to ingest.*

Burdock

Arctium lappa

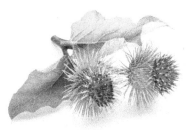

Medicinal parts used: root, leaves, seeds

I prefer to work with the root for food and medicine. The leaves are extremely bitter, and the seeds are surrounded by irritating hairs.

Properties: alterative, antibacterial, antifungal, anti-inflammatory, antimutagenic, cooling, demulcent, diaphoretic, diuretic, digestive bitter, emollient, grounding, kidney tonic, liver tonic, lymph tonic, nutritive, rejuvenating

Uses: Burdock root is an alterative, which means it is able to alter the body back to a state of health, especially with stubborn chronic conditions. It improves the health and function of the lymph, liver, kidneys, and digestive system. Burdock root works slowly yet effectively. Work with this root for at least 3 months before expecting to see changes in chronic health concerns. Burdock clears skin conditions, especially when they are dry, scaly, and inflamed, e.g., eczema, psoriasis, and chronic acne. Burdock supports optimal digestion and nutrient assimilation.

Common preparations: decoction, nourishing infusion, food, tincture, vinegar

Common dosage: Drink up to 1 quart of a burdock infusion, divided throughout the day, 1 to 3 times per week; consume 1 dropperful of tincture 3 times per day; or eat the root as a vegetable.

TIP: Burdock root contains up to 50 percent inulin, an insoluble and indigestible starch. Because it is insoluble, it will settle as a white sediment in the bottom of a burdock root tincture and vinegar. Inulin is healthy for the gut microbiome and can be included in your remedy.

Safety considerations: Burdock is a safe herb and nutritious food. Be cautious of the hairs that surround the seeds and cover the burrs. They are irritating to the skin. They can also irritate the lungs if they are breathed in.

Cinnamon

Cinnamomum zeylanicum, C. cassia

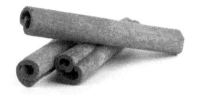

Medicinal part used: inner bark

Properties: antimicrobial, antispasmodic, astringent, circulation enhancer, demulcent, digestive, hypoglycemic, hypotensive, warming

Uses: Cinnamon fights bacteria, fungi, and viruses. It fights infections in the mouth, lungs, and throat while soothing mucous membranes. It is a warming herb that lowers blood pressure and increases circulation to the extremities, so it is especially helpful for people who have chills or chronically cold hands and feet. It improves digestive function and lowers blood sugar.

Common preparations: tisane, decoction, smoothie, food, elixir

Common dosage: You can consume 2 to 12 teaspoons of cinnamon powder as a therapeutic dose.

TIP: There are two species of cinnamon available on the market. One is cassia, *Cinnamomum cassia* (syn. *C. aromaticum*) and the other is Ceylon cinnamon, *Cinnamonum zeylanicum* (syn. *C. verum*). Ceylon cinnamon is thought to be sweeter and higher quality and is preferred. Cassia is what you'll probably see on grocery store spice shelves. They can be used interchangeably.

Safety considerations: In reasonable amounts, cinnamon is a safe herb. Its hypoglycemic and hypotensive properties mean it is best not to combine it with drugs with the same properties; it may increase their effects. Due to its volatile oil content, it can be harmful if used in amounts that drastically exceed therapeutic doses.

Comfrey

Symphytum x uplandicum

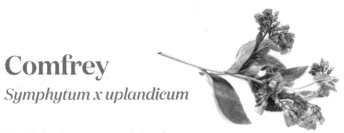

Medicinal parts used: leaf, root

Properties: demulcent, emollient, astringent, nutritive tonic, tissue repairing

Uses: Comfrey brings strength, flexibility, and nourishment to the mucous membranes of the respiratory, digestive, reproductive, and urinary systems. It heals damaged tissue of the skin, ligaments, tendons, and bones, giving them more strength and flexibility. Comfrey makes skin soft, flexible, and strong. Comfrey provides proteins that are found in short-term memory cells, improving their function. It offers a large range of minerals, vitamins, and proteins that support and improve overall health.

Common preparations: Dried leaf is consumed in infusions. The root and leaf are used in topical remedies.

Common dosage: For general health maintenance, consume up to 1 quart of a comfrey infusion, divided throughout the day, 1 day per week, or 2 to 4 times per week in acute situations for a maximum duration of 1 month.

> **TIP:** If you wish to grow comfrey, it should only be planted in a spot where it can live forever. Once it's planted, it will never be eradicated from that location. Any size piece of a comfrey root will grow a new plant. Do not disturb the soil around a comfrey plant or put live root pieces in your compost. Farm fields have been abandoned due to the accidental tilling and spreading of comfrey root pieces.

Safety considerations: Do not ingest comfrey root or fresh leaf. Dried leaves are safe in water infusions. Comfrey leaves can be confused with poisonous foxglove (Digitalis) leaves in the spring, so it is important to postpone harvest until comfrey is blooming and you know the plant well.

Elderflower and Elderberry

Sambucus nigra, S. canadensis

Medicinal parts used: flowers and berries

Properties: The flowers are antibacterial, anti-inflammatory, antiviral, calming, decongestant, diaphoretic, discutient, diuretic, emollient, and lymphagogue. The berries are anti-inflammatory, antioxidant, antiviral, immune supportive, diaphoretic, and diuretic.

Uses: Elderflowers relieve cold and flu symptoms. They clear mucous congestion in the sinuses and lungs. They cool a fever, although sometimes the fever will increase a little before it cools. Elderflower soothes the nerves, allowing restful sleep. As a mouthwash, it eases ulcers and inflamed gums. Elderberries support immune health by inhibiting viral replication. Berry preparations shorten influenza and herpes infection times. They help people who have tonsillitis, a cough, or ear congestion. They offer antioxidants that support eye and heart health. They decrease arthritis pain with their anti-inflammatory and diuretic properties.

Common preparations: The flowers are used in tisanes, honey, tinctures, elixirs, and food. The berries are used in decoctions, honey, syrups, tinctures, elixirs, oxymels, and shrubs.

Common dosage: Elderflower: Take 1 to 4 cups of tisane per day or as needed. Elderberry: Take 1 to 8 tablespoons of syrup or oxymel or 1 to 4 cups of tea per day or as needed. In cases of acute symptoms, take doses on the higher end of the range; for prevention, maintenance, or at the end of an illness, take lower doses.

TIP: Whole elderflowers make for tasty fritters when dipped in batter and panfried. Elderberries can be baked into fruit pies or crumbles. Fresh berry tinctures and syrups taste sweeter than dried berry preparations.

Safety considerations: Eating the raw berries, leaves, bark, or roots of elder shrub can cause nausea and vomiting. Only consume cooked or infused berries.

Ginger

Zingiber officinale

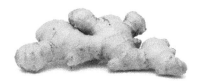

Medicinal part used: rhizome/root

Properties: antibacterial, antifungal, anti-inflammatory, antiparasitic, antiviral, carminative, circulatory enhancer, emmenagogue, expectorant, hypotensive

Uses: Ginger promotes circulation of the blood, warming chronically cold hands and feet. It is beneficial for heart health in general, helping modulate cholesterol levels and blood pressure. Ginger quells nausea, eases gas pains and cramping in the gut, relieves menstrual cramps, and uplifts the mood, relieving depression and anxiety. Ginger supports brain function and cognition. Ginger is anti-infective and helps break a fever. It is useful in cases of colds, flus, ear infections, respiratory infections, and intestinal infections.

Common preparations: tisane, tincture, syrup, elixir, spice blend, shrub

Common dosage: Any dose that works for you. If you take too much, it may become too spicy or heating. General dosage is 1 to 6 cups of tisane per day, 1 to 6 dropperfuls of tincture per day, or 1 to 6 teaspoons of syrup per day.

> **TIP:** Dried ginger is much more heating and pro-inflammatory than fresh ginger. I prefer to work with fresh ginger for this reason. I find it tastes better, is easy to find at the grocery store, and is less irritating than dried ginger.

Safety considerations: Ginger may have blood-thinning action, be an emmenagogue (stimulate menstrual bleeding), and potentially be inflammatory (as a rubefacient or irritating mouth mucosa).

Hawthorn

Crataegus species

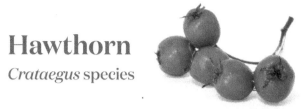

Medicinal parts used: berries, leaves, flowers

Properties: anti-inflammatory, astringent, calming, cardiac tonic, circulation enhancer, coronary and peripheral vasodilator, diuretic, hypotensive, nutritive, restorative

Uses: Hawthorn is best known as a heart tonic that supports and modulates the health of the cardiovascular system and blood pressure. It lowers cholesterol and prevents hardening of the arteries. It supports people who are heartbroken or grieving. It improves digestion, especially for people who are anxious. It soothes and calms the nerves and helps people sleep. Hawthorn improves cognition by increasing circulation of blood and oxygen to the brain. It aids healing after surgery and accelerates collagen generation.

Common preparations: tisane, decoction, nourishing infusion, syrup, vinegar, oxymel, tincture, elixir

Common dosage: Dose as needed and as feels right to you. Any dose is safe, due to its food-like nature. You can drink up to 1 quart of a hawthorn berry or leaf infusion per week, 1 to 6 dropperfuls of tincture per day, or 1 to 6 teaspoons of syrup per day.

> **TIP:** Hawthorn berry preparations taste delicious, especially with a little honey. The flowers and leaves are more astringent than the berries and have a hint of floral fruity undertones.

Safety considerations: Hawthorn is a safe, nourishing herb from the apple and rose family.

Lemon Balm

Melissa officinalis

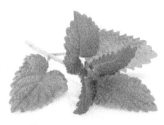

Medicinal parts used: leaves, flowers

Properties: anodyne, antidepressant, antihistamine, anti-inflammatory, anti-oxidant, antispasmodic, antiviral, anxiolytic, carminative, diaphoretic, hypotensive, immune supportive, nervine, sedative

Uses: Lemon balm supports the health of the nervous system by uplifting spirits and calming anxiety. It aids sleep and reduces pain. Its aromatic oils help soothe digestion and relax spasms in the gut and uterus. It can help prevent and treat diabetes by modulating blood sugar levels and oxidative stress. Lemon balm increases mental alertness and cognitive function, protecting against senility and mental decline. It is a tonic to the cardiovascular system and calms heart palpitations. Lemon balm is antibacterial and antiviral, specifically against herpes viruses. It relieves coughs, decongests, and opens the lungs. It supports people who have overactive thyroid. Lemon balm soothes skin irritations and slows skin aging.

Common preparations: tisane, honey, syrup, vinegar, oxymel, shrub, tincture, elixir

Common dosage: Take 2 to 6 cups of lemon balm tea or 2 to 6 dropperfuls of tincture per day or as needed. It can be applied topically to herpes sores.

TIP: Lemon balm is particularly attractive to bees. It releases the same pheromones that bees release when they are establishing a new home and organizing a colony. Lemon balm was traditionally rubbed on beehives to attract bees so they would nest there. Lemon balm is easy to grow and feeds the bees.

Safety considerations: Lemon balm is generally considered a safe herb, related to mint. It may exacerbate cases of underactive thyroid— hypothyroidism.

Linden

Tilia species

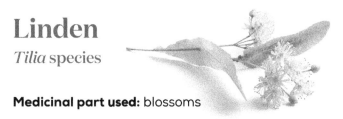

Medicinal part used: blossoms

Properties: antispasmodic, anti-inflammatory, anxiolytic, calming nervine, demulcent, diaphoretic, discutient, diuretic, emollient, heart tonic, hypotensive, nutritive, relaxant, sedative, sialagogue

Uses: Linden flowers have anti-inflammatory effects throughout the body. They support immune function, especially in cases of colds and flus. They reduce fevers, relieve coughs and hoarseness, soothe sore throats, and decongest sinuses and lungs. Linden protects the heart by reducing cholesterol, relaxing the arteries, and relieving stress. It is a heart tonic that helps restore health after heart attacks, strokes, or cardiovascular surgery. Linden soothes and calms the nervous system, especially for people who are overworked, frazzled, and stressed. Linden eases PMS symptoms and menstrual cramps. Linden's mucilage heals and restores the lining of the digestive tract.

Common preparations: infusion, tea, syrup, elixir, tincture

Common dosage: For an acute situation, take 3 to 8 cups of linden tea or infusion per day or 3 to 6 dropperfuls of tincture. For general health support, you can drink up 1 quart of linden infusion per week.

TIP: Linden flowers can make a rather thick tea; some people don't like the texture, though it is very healing to mucous membranes. To lessen the viscosity, drink the tea hot. Making a tea or infusion with whole linden blossoms yields a less glutinous drink than with cut-and-sifted blossoms. You can also make a nourishing herbal infusion with ½ ounce of linden flowers instead of the standard 1 ounce.

Safety considerations: Linden is considered a safe herb to consume.

Oat Straw
Avena sativa

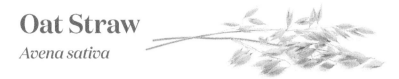

Medicinal parts used: stems, leaves, flowers, milky oat tops

Properties: adaptogen, antidepressant, anti-inflammatory, antispasmodic, aphrodisiac, carminative, demulcent, diaphoretic, diuretic, emollient, febrifuge, nervine, nutritive tonic, restorative, vulnerary, revitalizing

Uses: Oat straw nourishes and builds health, especially for folks with chronic health conditions and general debility. It nourishes and tones the nervous system. It is especially suited for people who are stressed, overworked, frazzled, or anxious. Oat straw both builds energy and allows restful sleep. It improves synaptic functioning and communication between nerves. Oat straw improves the integrity of the bones, joints, hair, teeth, nails, and skin. It improves the functioning of the entire cardiovascular system. Oat straw also improves fertility and sexual vitality.

Common preparations: nourishing herbal infusion, tincture, tea

Common dosage: For general health maintenance, take 1 to 2 quarts of oat-straw infusion per week, 2 to 6 dropperfuls of tincture (milky oat tops) per day or as needed for acute situations, and 2 to 6 cups of decoction per day or as you like.

TIP: Tincture made from the fresh milky oat tops has a stronger sedative action than the infusion of oat straw. The oat straw is more for minerals and overall health.

Safety considerations: Oat straw is a safe, nourishing herb. Be cautious if you have a gluten allergy. Oats are not known to have gluten, but they may be processed in a facility with gluten-containing grains. Moderate amounts of oat straw are safe for people with gluten intolerance and celiac disease.

Red Clover

Trifolium pratense

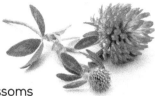

Medicinal part used: blossoms

Properties: alterative, anticancer, anti-inflammatory, antispasmodic, expectorant, astringent, discutient, digestive tonic, hormone modulator, respiratory tonic, reproductive tonic, nutritive

Uses: Red clover nourishes the entire body with an array of vitamins and minerals. Red clover blossoms improve the health of the blood, bones, skin, lymph, lungs, endocrine glands, and reproductive organs. It improves skin troubled by eczema and acne. It cools inflamed lungs and stops coughing. Red clover's discutient action helps soften, shrink, or dissolve hard swellings and cysts. Red clover soothes the nerves and emotions, stabilizes the mind, and eases anxiety. Red clover helps lymph move and improves the functioning of the body's immune response.

Common preparation: infusion

Common dosage: Take 1 to 2 quarts of red clover infusion per week.

TIP: Even though red clover has constituents that thin blood, it also has constituents with an opposite effect, typically yielding an overall balancing effect, especially when consumed as an infusion. Red clover is often thought to contain estrogen that causes an undesirable increase of estrogen in the body. It doesn't contain estrogen. Instead, it provides phytosterols ("plant hormones") that human gut flora can change into constituents that act in the body like a mild form of estrogen. Consequently, it has an overall modulating effect on estrogen in the body, increasing and blocking its effects when needed.

Safety considerations: Red clover is a safe, nourishing herb. It has potential to thin the blood and may add to the effect of pharmaceutical blood thinners when ingested in capsules, standardized extracts, and supplements. See the tip above for more info.

Rose

Rosa species

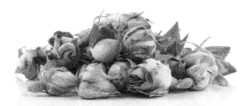

Medicinal parts used: hips, petals, flower buds

Properties: The hips are anti-inflammatory, antimutagenic, antioxidant, diuretic, nutritive tonic, and revitalizing. The petals and flower buds are analgesic, anti-infective, anti-inflammatory, antioxidant, antispasmodic, astringent, calming, tonic, nervine, and sedative.

Uses: Rose hips support the cardiovascular system by strengthening the heart, improving circulation, and helping prevent arteriosclerosis. They increase immune defense against bacterial and viral infections; support digestion and relieve constipation; and improve kidney and bladder health. Rose petals and flower buds support and nourish the heart, stomach, liver, lungs, and reproductive system. They soothe and calm digestive distress; relieve coughs and congestion; support immune defense by moving lymph and cooling fevers; promote calm and relaxation; and improve skin health. They relieve a broad range of female reproductive system complaints that are connected to hormone fluctuations.

Common preparations: The hips are used in syrups, jellies and jams, food, tisanes, decoctions, infusions, smoothies, and vinegar. Petals and flower buds are used in tisanes, syrups, jellies and jams, food, vinegar, oxymels, shrubs, honey, tinctures, and elixirs.

Common dosage: Take 3 to 6 cups of rose tea a day; 1 to 3 dropperfuls of tincture 3 to 6 times a day; or 3 to 6 teaspoons of syrup, oxymel, vinegar, or elixir a day.

TIP: Roses that are highly aromatic are best to use. Do not use roses from florists because they are sprayed with herbicides, fungicides, and pesticides. *Rosa rugosa* is my favorite rose to grow and forage, with large, fragrant flowers and plump, fleshy hips.

Safety considerations: Rose petals and hips are both safe, nourishing herbs.

Schisandra

Schisandra chinensis

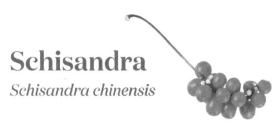

Medicinal part used: berries

Properties: adaptogen, antiasthmatic, anti-inflammatory, antioxidant, anxiolytic, astringent, expectorant, immune tonic, kidney tonic, liver protective, nervine

Uses: Schisandra is a nourishing adaptogen that offers whole-body health. Adaptogens are herbs that are nontoxic and nonspecific in action and that normalize body functions. Schisandra has protective actions on the liver, lungs, heart, and gut. It increases mental clarity, relieves anxiety, and builds resilience to stress. It increases sexual vitality, reduces fatigue, and relieves insomnia. It modulates blood pressure and reduces heart palpitations.

Common preparations: tisane, infusion, tincture, elixir, syrup, honey, smoothie

Common dosage: You can consume 3 cups of schisandra tisane or 1 to 3 dropperfuls of tincture a day, or up to 1 quart of schisandra infusion per week.

TIP: Schisandra is called "the five-flavor fruit." It contains all five flavors: bitter, sweet, pungent, salty, and sour. Its strong and unique flavor is best enjoyed in small amounts. When you make an infusion with the berries, they do not need to be strained out. They will settle to the bottom of the jar and you can drink the infusion off the top, straining them through your teeth as you get to the bottom. The infusion can be frozen into pink ice cubes and then put into water or drinks to add flavor as they melt.

Safety considerations: Schisandra is a safe, nourishing herb.

Stinging Nettle
Urtica dioica

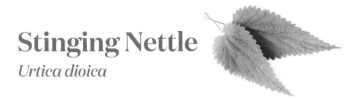

Medicinal parts used: leaves and stems harvested before flowering

Properties: adaptogen, alterative, antihistamine, anti-inflammatory, diuretic, expectorant, general tonic, kidney tonic, lymphagogue, nutritive, restorative

Uses: Stinging nettle offers increased energy and nutrition. It builds, strengthens, and restores health throughout the body. If you are not sure what herb to take for a condition, consider nettle. It could likely help! Notably, nettle tones and restores health to the kidneys and the adrenals. It is a remedy for allergy symptoms and will eventually eliminate them if consumed for a year. Nettle has an affinity for the lungs, bringing them strength and flexibility. The mineral content in nettle builds bones, tones skin, strengthens nails, brings shine to hair, and offers an overall healthy glow to a person.

Common preparations: infusion, vinegar, food

Common dosage: 1 to 2 quarts of stinging nettle infusion per week

TIP: Stinging nettle infusions taste very green. If you are not used to consuming green foods, the chlorophyll may make you feel a little nauseous. Drinking a watered-down infusion will help, and you can then work your way up to full strength. Drinking an infusion over ice also cuts the green flavor. Warming the nettle infusion with some miso paste is another way to change the flavor and make it more palatable.

Safety considerations: Stinging nettle is a safe, nourishing herb. However, if you touch or brush against the living or fresh plant, it will sting you, leaving a rash that resembles hives. Protect your skin with gloves and long sleeves when harvesting or working with fresh nettle leaf.

Tulsi (Holy Basil)

Ocimum tenuiflorum

Medicinal parts used: leaves, flowers

Properties: adaptogen, analgesic, anticoagulant, antidepressant, antimicrobial, antioxidant, antiseptic, antispasmodic, anxiolytic, aromatic, cardiovascular tonic, carminative, diaphoretic, diffusive, digestive, galactagogue, hypoglycemic, liver tonic, nervine

Uses: Tulsi offers an array of benefits throughout the body. It is an adaptogen. Adaptogen herbs are nontoxic and nonspecific in action and normalize body functions. Tulsi modulates and supports immune functions. It is effective against colds and flus. It eases anxiety, calms the nerves, and builds resilience to stress. It centers the mind and aids in concentration and meditation. It clears brain fog, enhances circulation, and relieves inflammation and pain. Tulsi supports digestion, quells heartburn and nausea, and slows gut transit time.

Common preparations: tisane, honey, tincture, elixir, oxymel, shrub

Common dosage: Take 1 to 3 cups of tisane a day, 3 to 6 dropperfuls of tincture a day, or 1 to 3 teaspoons of oxymel a day.

TIP: Also known as holy basil, tulsi is a sacred plant seen as the embodiment of the Divine Mother on Earth. It is planted in places of honor, outside homes and temples. There are multiple varieties of tulsi that have different flavors but can be used interchangeably for the recipes in this book.

Safety considerations: Tulsi, a species of basil, is a safe herb. It is mildly anticoagulant. Caution is advised if using blood-thinning pharmaceuticals. Tulsi can lower blood sugar, so use caution if taking insulin and blood sugar–lowering pharmaceuticals. Tulsi may lower fertility for men and women while taking it but not long-term.

Where to Get Your Herbs

You can procure your herbs in a few ways. You can grow them yourself; forage them; or purchase them from local herb shops, health-food stores, herb farms, or online distributors. The Resources section (see page 169) contains a list of reliable retailers. Increasingly, pharmacies and big-box stores stock the more common medicinal herbs, too.

It is recommended to source organically grown herbs when possible. This is to avoid pesticide residue or synthetic fertilizers in your medicine. Organically grown herbs are better not only for your health but also for the health of the environment.

Purchase quality herbs that have bright color and fresh scent and flavor. Aromatic herbs are best used within a year of harvest. Over time, their volatile oils dissipate, and they lose their flavor, scent, and medicine. Mineral-rich herbs can be stored longer. Always store herbs away from sunlight.

Growing Your Own Herbs

When you grow your own herbs, you learn about the plants as you tend them. Growing your own herbs saves money and provides the best-quality plants to make medicine with.

You can grow herbs in pots on your apartment balcony or in a small backyard herb garden. To grow herbs in pots, fill them with a combination of potting soil and compost. Plant seeds, annual seedlings, or small perennials. Most herbs prefer warm sunny locations. Pots dry out quickly and need to be watered daily or whenever the soil is dry.

A small backyard garden will need to be dug, clearing away the lawn. Add compost, then plant seeds, annual seedlings, and perennial plants. Weeding the grass and undesired plants as the garden grows is important to provide space and nutrients to the herbs you planted. If deer live around you, you may need to put up a fence to protect your garden from them.

In northern climates, annuals will die in the winter and perennials will come back the following spring. Herbs that are easy to grow in both pots and gardens include rosemary, calendula, tulsi, chamomile, mint, thyme, fennel, lemon balm, and comfrey. If you have extra space, you can plant medicinal trees and shrubs, such as linden, elder, and hawthorn. Many wild herbs can be grown easily in pots and in the garden. In fact, they are often the weeds that show up on their own. These plants are easy to forage from your own backyard or vacant city lots.

DRYING YOUR OWN HERBS

The recipes in this book are made with either fresh or dried herbs. If you are growing or foraging your own herbs, you may want to dry them to preserve them for future tisanes and infusions.

It is best to harvest herbs when they are free of moisture. Ideally, it has not rained for 48 hours prior to harvest time. Harvest herbs in the middle of the day after the morning dew has dried and before the evening dew sets in. Once your herbs are harvested, keep them away from sunlight while they are drying and when they are stored.

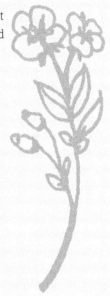

Dry your herbs in a room with good air circulation and low humidity. Herbs can be dried in multiple ways. The stems can be tied together in small bundles and hung upside down. They can be spread out on screens or in open flat baskets, which works well for leaves and flowers that are not on stems. The screens can be propped up on blocks, so that air flows under them as well as over them. If you have small amounts of herbs to dry, you can dry them in a dehydrator on low heat or in brown paper bags that are lightly shaken several times per day.

Foraging for Herbs

Foraging refers to harvesting wild plants for medicine or food. For the beginner herbalist, stick to harvesting common herbs that grow in your own backyard, garden, or neighborhood farm. Common herbs to get to know include dandelion, burdock, goldenrod, linden, hawthorn, rose, elder, yarrow, and hypericum. Only harvest herbs that you are 100 percent sure you can identify and whose specific population you have watched for a full year prior to harvesting. Foraging is not something to be taken lightly or done on a whim.

Wild foraging beyond familiar backyard plants is for the advanced herbalist who can identify plants with 100 percent accuracy. They must also have knowledge of and be able to identify poisonous plants that grow in the area. They must also be aware of what pollution may be in the soil.

A forager needs to understand the life cycle of the plant, the part of the plant they are harvesting, and the effect that part has on maintaining the plant population. When harvesting the seeds from an annual plant, they must know to leave seeds for future growth. If harvesting a root, they need to understand that they are killing the plant and possibly reducing the plant population.

Ultimately, if you want to harvest your own herbs, it is best to grow them and to "weed" them from your own garden, community garden plot, or potted balcony garden.

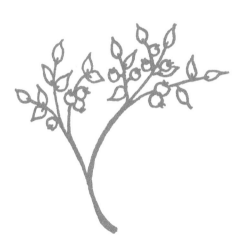

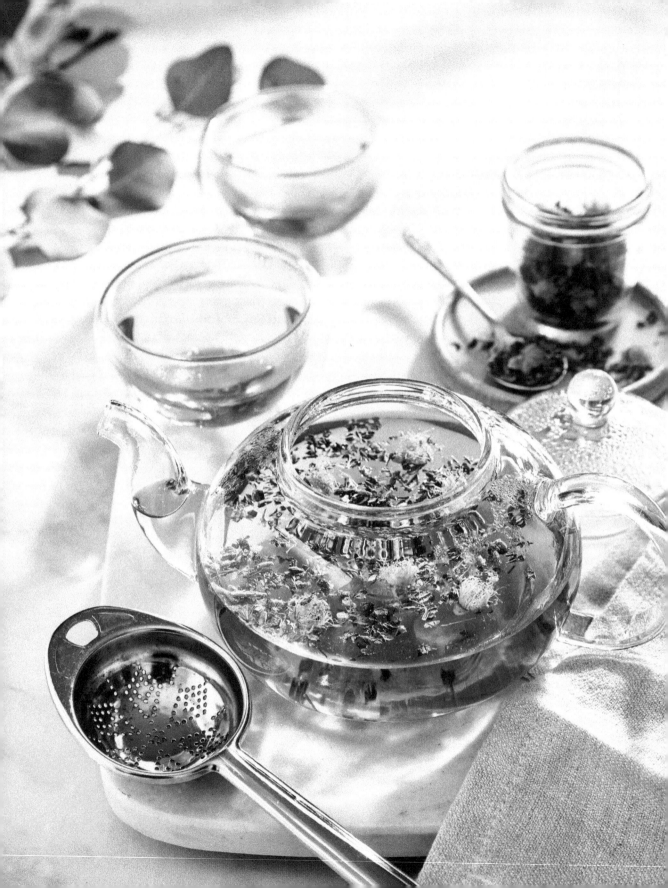

CHAPTER 3

How to Prepare Herbal Beverages

The home herbalist can make medicinal herbal preparations in their own kitchen with herbs they purchase or grow and a few staple pantry items. Although herbal preparations can be used topically and internally, one of the easiest and most enjoyable ways to reap their benefits is by making and consuming healing herbal drinks.

All the recipes in this book build and improve health with the nutrients and medicinal constituents extracted from herbs. This chapter provides useful information about the types of drinks you'll find in the recipe chapters, including infusions, tisanes, tinctures, honies, syrups, shrubs, and oxymels. You'll also learn tips for labeling, storing, and dispensing the recipes that you make.

Types of Drinkable Herbal Infusions

When people think of a drinkable herbal infusion, they likely imagine an herbal tea made with boiling water. However, herbs can be infused in a variety of liquids that will extract their medicinal constituents. Herbalists call these solvent liquids the *menstruum*. The menstruums we work with in this book include water, honey, alcohol, and vinegar. The herb that is being infused is called the *marc*.

Once an herb-infused menstruum is made, it can either stand alone as a beverage or be added to a base such as water, juice, smoothies, bubbly water, cocktails, or mocktails.

Tisanes, Infusions, and Decoctions

Extracting the healing properties of herbs into water is the oldest and most common way to make healing herbal drinks. Water extracts a wide variety of nourishing and medicinal constituents from plants, including vitamins, minerals, bitter substances, mucilage, antioxidants, and volatile oils. These drinks are easy and quick to prepare. The three ways to extract herbs into water are tisanes, infusions, and decoctions.

TISANES

You can think of a tisane as an herbal tea that is quick to make, usually only requiring 20 minutes to steep in hot water. Tisanes are made using a small amount of fresh or dried medicinal herb and the preparation method that harnesses the water-soluble medicinal constituents and the volatile oils from the herbs. The herbs in a tisane are measured by the teaspoon, tablespoon, or cup. A simple tisane to try is Summer Blossom Nervine Tisane (page 105).

It's worth noting that a tisane is distinct from caffeinated tea. Technically the word "tea" refers to drinks containing the plant *Camellia sinensis*, which is what black, green, and white teas are made from.

INFUSIONS

An infusion is similar to a tisane; however, infusions require a larger amount of herbs to be steeped for at least 4 hours. The herbs used contain a higher quantity of vitamins, minerals, protein, and other health-building nutrients, which take longer to extract. Infusions are never made with aromatic herbs. A superb infusion is Calming Oat Straw Infusion (page 123).

You will sometimes see herbalists refer to infusions by the full name of "nourishing herbal infusions," but in this book, we will simply call them infusions.

DECOCTIONS

Decoctions are how we make tea from tough plant parts like roots, barks, seeds, berries, lichens, and mushrooms. Due to their tough nature, it takes more heat and agitation to extract the medicinal constituents and nutrients into water. Accordingly, a decoction is made by simmering the plant material in water, usually for around 20 to 60 minutes. The Echinacea and Elderberry Immune Defense Decoction (page 48) is a tasty immune-building remedy to start with.

Honey Infusions

As you might expect, these are made by infusing herbs in honey. Not only does this allow you to enjoy the medicinal properties of the herbs, but you can also reap the natural benefits of honey, which is known to soothe sore throats and coughs, hydrate tissues, and promote anti-bacterial activity.

Herbal honey can be made with fresh or dried herbs. Honey is hydrophilic, which means it draws water out of fresh herbs along with some of their medicinal constituents. After infusing fresh herbs in honey for a few days, the herbs shrink in size as the honey extracts all the herbs' water content. A great recipe to start with is the Cooling Rose Petal Honey (page 88).

Herb-Infused Syrups

Syrups are another satisfyingly sweet way to take herbal medicine. Syrups are made by heavily sweetening a concentrated decoction or tisane with honey or sugar. These syrups can add flavor and medicine to beverages. They are also a nice way to administer herbs to children. Elderberry Antiviral Syrup (page 49) is a good immune-supportive syrup to start with.

Tinctures (Alcohol Infusions)

A tincture is made by infusing medicinal herbs in alcohol. Tinctures are the strongest infusions and are often used for medicinal purposes because alcohol is especially effective at extracting and concentrating the medicinal constituents of herbs, rather than the vitamins and minerals.

Tinctures are commonly used for acute health concerns such as infections, digestive distress, or insomnia. They can also be used for tonic effects that strengthen and improve the health of specific organs and body systems. For example, St. John's Wort Tincture to Ease Nerve Pain (page 109) is specific to healing nerve damage and pain. Tinctures are taken in small doses, either by drops, dropperfuls, milliliters, or teaspoons.

You will come across some tinctures in this book known as bitters, which are tinctures made with bitter, sour, and aromatic herb combinations to improve the health of the digestive system. One example of a bitters recipe is Premeal Dandelion, Orange, and Fennel Bitters (page 66).

You will also find some tinctures called elixirs, which are tinctures that have been sweetened. I often sweeten tinctures with either plain or herb-infused honey. I like to make elixirs with tonic herbs (herbs used for a specific purpose and taken regularly over a longer period of time), an example of which is the Rose Petal Elixir for Reproductive Health (page 93).

The final tincture you will see in the book is cordials, which are elixirs that are specific for heart health, such as the Herbal Cordial for Cardiac Protection (page 144).

Vinegar Infusions

Herbal vinegar infusions are made in the same way as tinctures but using vinegar instead of alcohol. They are technically called "aceta" or an "acetum" but are commonly called herbal vinegars. Vinegar is a solvent that extracts vitamins, minerals, and some medicinal constituents from plants. Vinegar infusions are lovely to have in the kitchen to use as a condiment or base for marinades and salad dressings. They can also be added to drinks.

I prefer apple cider vinegar, but any vinegar other than white vinegar will do. Before infusing herbs into vinegar, it is best to pasteurize it to extend the herbal vinegar's shelf life. Without pasteurization, there could be an unwanted reaction between the live colonies of microbes in the vinegar and the ones on the fresh plant material. You can find how to pasteurize vinegar in the recipes in this book, such as in the Dandelion Vinegar for Skin and Hair Enrichment (page 81).

Aside from herbal vinegars, this book also contains vinegar-based herbal drinks called oxymels and shrubs. An oxymel is made with a combination of herbs, apple cider vinegar, and honey. Oxymels can be taken by the spoonful or shot glass or added to drinks. On page 159, you will find the Antioxidant Oxymel with Rosemary and Thyme. An herbal shrub is made with herbs, vinegar, fruit, and a sweetener such as sugar or honey. Shrubs can be enjoyed in small amounts or added to drinks. A delicious one to try is the Ginger-Blueberry Shrub for Better Digestion (page 63).

Storing, Labeling, and Dispensing Your Infusions

Once your herb-infused remedy is made, you will need to store it. Remedies can be stored in a variety of ways. Mason jars of various sizes work well, and you can pour your remedy from them into smaller-dosage bottles. Recycled baby-food jars and vinegar bottles work well, too.

Boston round amber bottles are useful to store tinctures, elixirs, oxymels, shrubs, and syrups. You can find them online or at your local herb shop. If making a tincture, store it in a Boston round amber bottle with a dropper top for easy administering. However, don't store tinctures for extended periods of time in bottles with rubber dropper caps. The alcohol evaporates into the rubber dropper top, eroding the rubber and evaporating through it. This makes the remedy taste like rubber and reduces the amount left in the bottle as it evaporates. The bottles can be sealed with normal lids and the dropper lids kept on the side to be used as needed.

Dried herbs and tea blends can be stored in glass jars, resealable plastic food bags, brown paper bags designed for storing tea, or brown paper lunch bags.

It is handy to keep dropper tops, teaspoons, small measuring cups, shot glasses, cordial glasses, and bottles that pour on hand for measuring and administering your herbal preparations.

Make sure to label all your remedies. Label the containers that they infuse in and then label the final bottles and jars they are strained over. It is very hard to recognize herbs once they have been infusing in the menstruum (solvent) for a long time. You may think you'll remember what herb is in there or the day the remedies were made, but you likely won't. On the labels, include the date the remedy was made, the name of the herb, the part of the herb, the menstruum (solvent) used, and the suggested dosage or use. It is especially important to put detailed labels on any preparations that you plan to give to anyone else.

Herbal remedies made with water are best stored in the refrigerator and will last 1 to 5 days. Remedies made with honey and vinegar can last for 1 to 3 years or even longer, especially if they are made with pasteurized vinegar and stored in a cool place. Remedies made with alcohol can last for 20 years or more. It is best to store unrefrigerated herbal remedies in a cool dark cabinet away from direct sunlight and heat to increase their shelf life and retain their quality. I have been conservative with the storage times. My hope is that you will use up the remedies before their suggested expiration dates, which are not hard and fast. Use your nose in addition to checking the bottle labels; if the remedy smells good, it's likely still good.

SALVES, OILS, CREAMS

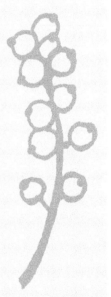

Herbs improve health not only from the inside out but also from the outside in. They can be made into a variety of topical preparations to soothe, mend, and heal problems of the skin. Topical preparations can help ease external and internal aches, pains, and inflammations as well. These preparations can be as simple as applying an herbal tea, infusion, or tincture topically. Other preparations include herb-infused oils, which can be made with any pure oil such as olive, almond, sesame, or coconut. Dry or fresh herbs are infused into the oil, often with a gentle heat. They are then strained and applied straight or combined with various ingredients to create other topical remedies. Herb-infused oils combined with beeswax make salves. When oils are combined with tallow or solid plant fats, e.g., shea butter, they create rich creams. Infused oils combined with teas and solid fats create lotions.

Herb-infused oils made with dried herbs can be used internally when cooking food, but they aren't added to drinks, so we don't cover them in this book. If you're interested in learning more about herb-infused oils, check the Resources section (see page 169).

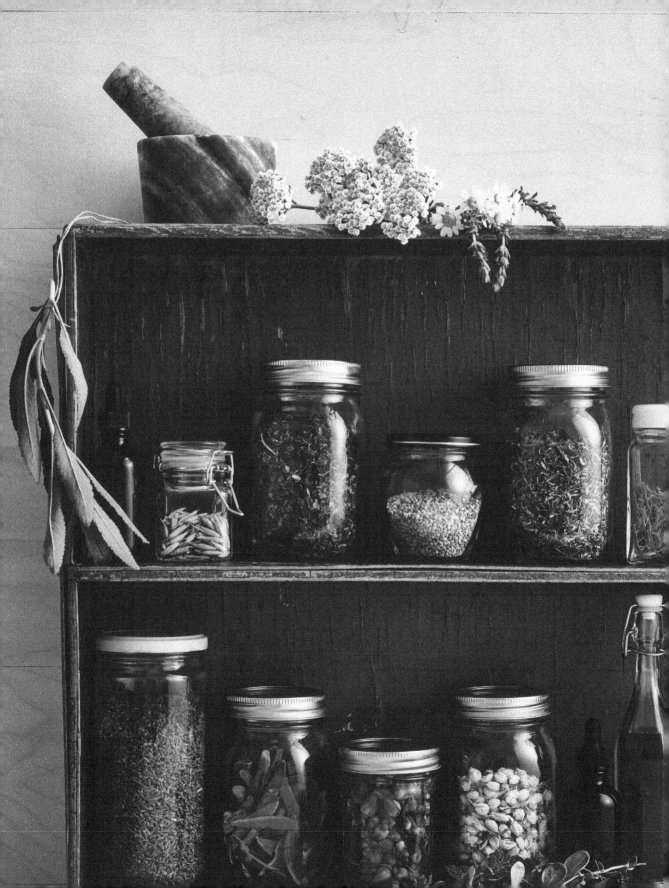

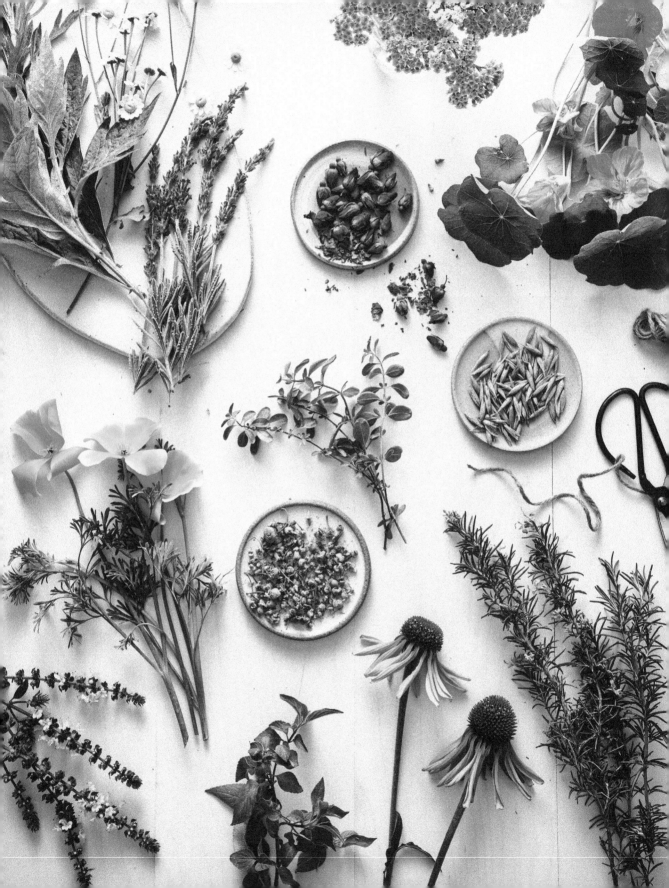

PART II

Healing Herbal Infusions

Making herb-infused drinks is a creative process, similar to cooking a healthy meal. The chapters to come highlight body systems and offer recipes that address a variety of health concerns in each of those systems. Most of the recipes in this book contain one to three herbs to make it easy for you to source the ingredients and make the healing beverages.

Making "simples" (remedies made using a single herb) gives us a clear understanding of each herb we work with, which allows us to share precise information about the herbs with our friends and family. Once you get the hang of basic techniques and learn about a core group of herbs, you can start to experiment and play with recipes to find the flavors and grouped effects that work best for you and those you make remedies for. Making healing herbal drinks is a fun and playful process where art and science meet to create health-promoting remedies.

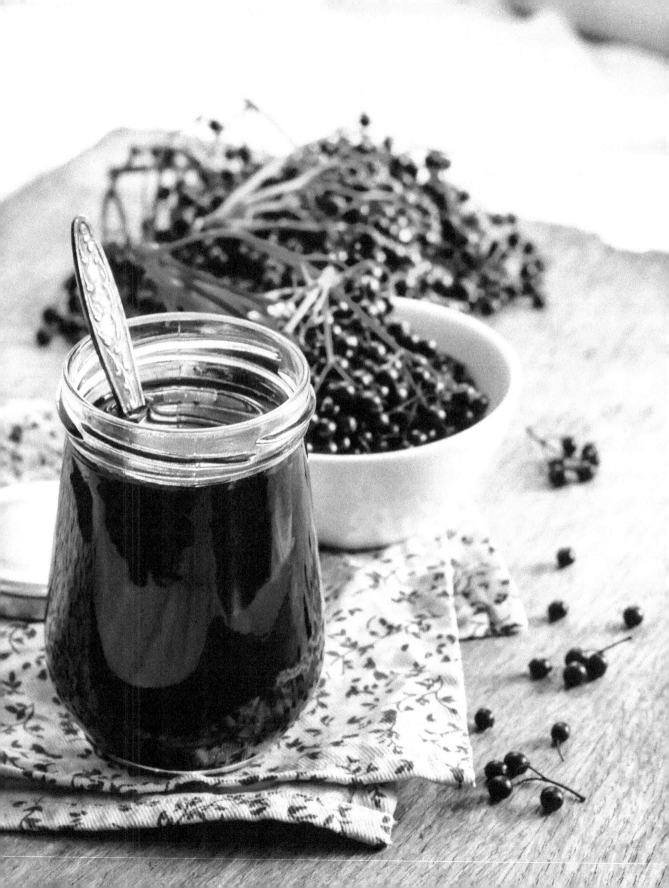

For the Immune System

The immune system runs throughout the body. The lymphatic system carries immune cells around the body. The digestive tract and lungs are lined with immune cells, protecting the body where the outside world first makes contact with the inside world. There are two aspects to the immune system: innate immunity and adaptive immunity. Innate immunity protects us from pathogens (disease-causing organisms) and mutated cells with its variety of immune cells and the microbiome. (The microbiome is the colony of living bacteria and yeast in the gut with which we have a mutually beneficial relationship.) Adaptive immunity protects our body with antibodies it learned to make after initial exposure to foreign substances such as bacteria, viruses, and allergens.

Autoimmune conditions and chronic inflammations happen when the immune system is not functioning well. It could be overworked, undernourished, exhausted, or stressed. Herbs support immune functions in a variety of ways. They have constituents that kill pathogens or interfere with their replication. They nourish and restore health and homeostasis (the body's ability to maintain a stable internal environment) to various aspects of the immune response, working to reverse chronic immune depletion, inflammation, and overreactions.

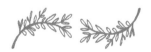

Immune-Tune Astragalus Infusion

MAKES: 4 cups

Astragalus root is an adaptogen, which is a substance that works to support body systems, resist stress, and build energy so we can ward off disease and maintain health. This infusion is especially helpful if you feel weak or are in recovery from a virus, disease, or other health problem. You may incorporate the infusion as a daily or weekly drink during the cold and flu season or if you live in an area with ticks and Lyme disease. The root makes for an enjoyable infusion with its sweet, earthy taste.

1 ounce astragalus root, cut and sifted	4 cups boiling water	Honey, for serving (optional)

1. Put the astragalus root in a 32-ounce mason jar, then fill the jar to the top with the boiling water. Cover with a tight lid, and steep for a minimum of 4 hours or up to overnight.

2. Line the mouth of a ceramic drip coffee filter with a straining cloth. Pour the infusion through the filter into a clean 32-ounce mason jar.

3. Gather the corners of the straining cloth, and wring the cloth to squeeze as much liquid from the herbs as you can.

4. Stir in honey to taste, if desired. You can drink the infusion from the jar or by the mug. Store any remaining infusion in a covered jar in the refrigerator for up to 2 days.

NOTE: You can freeze the infusion in ice cube trays and use when cooking rice, soup, or vegetables. You can also add this infusion to smoothies, such as Immune Defense Herbal Smoothie with Berries (page 52).

Immune-Boosting Nettle-Miso Broth

MAKES: 4 cups

This nourishing broth is rich in protein and minerals and is a healthy soup to serve your family and friends. You can also sip on this broth when you need an immune boost or are too sick to eat solid food. It is easy to digest, improves the health of the microbiome, and supports immunity by providing necessary nutrition.

1 ounce stinging nettle leaf	4 cups boiling water 2 tablespoons miso	Tamari, for serving (optional)

1. Put the nettle leaf in a 32-ounce mason jar, then fill the jar to the top with the boiling water. Cover with a tight lid, and steep for a minimum of 4 hours or up to overnight.

2. Line the mouth of a ceramic drip coffee filter with a straining cloth. Pour the infusion through the filter into a clean 32-ounce mason jar.

3. Gather the corners of the straining cloth, and wring the cloth to squeeze as much liquid from the herbs as you can.

4. Pour the infusion into a saucepot, and heat without bringing to a boil.

5. Hold a tea strainer over the pot. Using the back of a spoon, press the miso through the strainer into the pot.

6. Stir in tamari to taste, if desired. Remove from the heat.

7. Pour the nettle-miso broth into a large mug, and enjoy as a warm sipping broth. Store any remaining infusion in a covered jar in the refrigerator for up to 2 days.

NOTE: Miso is a fermented bean paste that not only adds umami flavor to food but also supports immune-system health due to its probiotic content, shortening infection and recovery times. It also benefits the digestive, cardiovascular, and reproductive systems and mental health.

Catnip and Elderflower Tisane to Ease Fever and Coughs

MAKES: 4 cups

This tisane has a light mint and sweet floral taste. It is beneficial for adults and children when they need to reduce a fever or ease a cough. Both catnip and elderflower soothe irritability and agitation. They are calming and allow restful sleep, which is helpful when you have a fever.

2 tablespoons dried catnip leaf or ¼ cup fresh

2 tablespoons dried elderflower or ¼ cup fresh

4 cups boiling water
Honey, for serving (optional)

1. Put the catnip and elderflower in a teapot, then cover with the boiling water. Cover with a lid, and steep for 20 minutes.

2. Pour the tisane through a tea strainer into a clean 32-ounce mason jar.

3. Sweeten with honey to taste, if desired. Enjoy the tisane straight from the jar, or pour into a mug to drink. Store any remaining tisane in a covered jar in the refrigerator for up to 2 days.

NOTE: You can also pour this tisane into a thermos to keep it warm and sip on throughout the day.

Echinacea and Elderberry Immune Defense Decoction

MAKES: 4 cups

This infused drink will really get your immune system working. Echinacea increases white blood cell activity to hunt pathogens and fight infections. Elderberry inhibits viral replication. Cinnamon adds warming spice and increases blood circulation and warmth throughout the body. You can drink this decoction frequently throughout the day at the onset of a cold or flu or if you have been exposed.

2 tablespoons dried echinacea root

2 tablespoons dried elderberries

1 teaspoon cinnamon chips or ½ cinnamon stick

5 cups water

Honey or preferred sweetener, for serving (optional)

1. In a saucepot, combine the echinacea, elderberries, and cinnamon. Cover with the water. Bring to a boil.

2. Reduce the heat to a simmer. Simmer for 30 minutes. Remove from the heat.

3. Pour the decoction through a tea strainer into a clean 32-ounce mason jar.

4. Sweeten with honey, if desired. Enjoy the decoction straight from the jar, or drink by the mug. Store any remaining decoction in a covered jar in the refrigerator for up to 2 days.

NOTE: Instead of cinnamon, you can add 1 teaspoon of dried hibiscus flowers to the pot for a hint of sourness.

Elderberry Antiviral Syrup

MAKES: 4 cups

Have this syrup on hand to keep viral infections at bay, especially through the winter. Taking elderberry syrup at the onset of a viral infection has been shown to reduce the time span of the infection, leading to a faster recovery. Add this tasty syrup to bubbly water, smoothies (such as Immune Defense Herbal Smoothie with Berries, page 52), or tea or enjoy by the spoonful. At the first hint of a viral infection, take a spoonful every 1 to 2 hours, or put 8 tablespoons in a water bottle or thermos and sip throughout the day.

4 cups dried elderberries or 8 cups fresh or frozen

8 cups water

2 cups honey or sugar

1. Put the elderberries in a soup pot, and cover with the water. Bring to a boil.

2. Reduce the heat to a simmer. Simmer until the liquid has reduced by half. Remove from the heat.

3. Line the mouth of a ceramic drip coffee filter with a straining cloth. Pour the decoction through the filter into a clean 32-ounce mason jar.

4. Gather the corners of the straining cloth, and wring the cloth to squeeze as much liquid from the berries as you can.

5. Stir the honey into the warm decoction until dissolved. Cover the jar tightly, label, and store in the refrigerator for up to 6 months.

NOTE: Elderberries are high in pectin. Sometimes the pectin will turn the syrup a little gloppy. Warming spices, such as ginger, cinnamon, and cloves, are often added to elderberry syrup. You can do this, too, but first try the plain elderberry taste and strength.

Viral Protection Elderberry Tincture

MAKES: 2 cups

Elderberry tinctures can help prevent a cold or flu from taking hold and provide immune support if one does. Elderberries inhibit viral replication so your immune system can clear the virus faster. Fresh or frozen elderberries make for a delicious tincture. It can also be made with dried elderberries, which are easy to purchase in bulk.

2 cups fresh elderberries or 1 cup dried

1½ cups 100-proof vodka

1. Put the elderberries in a clean 16-ounce mason jar, then fill the jar with the vodka. Cover with a tight lid, label, and let infuse for 6 weeks away from direct sunlight.

2. Line the mouth of a ceramic drip coffee filter with a straining cloth. Pour the tincture through the filter into a clean 32-ounce mason jar.

3. Gather the corners of the straining cloth, and wring the cloth to squeeze as much liquid from the berries as you can.

4. Pour the tincture through a small funnel into 4 clean (4-ounce) Boston round amber bottles. Cover with tight lids, and label. Tinctures keep indefinitely due to their alcohol content.

NOTE: This tincture can be taken by the teaspoon, tablespoon, or ounce as needed. It can be added to bubbly or plain water, tea, or juice for an immune-supporting beverage.

Health-Promoting Elderberry-Ginger Mocktail

MAKES: 2 cups

This is a fun and tasty elderberry drink that is lovely to share with friends or bring to a holiday gathering. It is a great option if you are avoiding alcohol but still want to drink a cocktail-like beverage. Even better is that this drink is good for you. Adding a shot glass of elderberry tincture turns it into a health-promoting mocktail. This recipe uses syrups and tinctures that you can make at home or purchase.

1 ounce Elderberry Antiviral Syrup (page 49)

½ ounce Ginger Syrup to Ease an Upset Stomach (page 62)

1 ounce Viral Protection Elderberry Tincture (page 50) (optional)

1¾ cups bubbly water

Ice, for serving

Lime wedge, for serving

1. Pour the elderberry syrup and ginger syrup into a pint glass.

2. Add the elderberry tincture, if desired.

3. Fill the glass with the bubbly water and ice.

4. Squeeze in the juice from a lime wedge, or leave the wedge as a garnish on the rim of the glass.

NOTE: You can leave out the ginger syrup if you do not want the spicy heat it offers. Add a splash of lemonade to add sweet and sour citrus flavor.

Immune Defense Herbal Smoothie with Berries

MAKES: 4 cups

This smoothie contains astragalus root and rose hips, which both nourish the immune system. With the addition of elderberry syrup, this smoothie builds the body's immune defense against viruses. Drink this smoothie during the cold and flu season to increase your resistance to infections. It is tasty and nourishing for kids and adults alike. Astragalus has a sweet, earthy flavor, and rose hips and elderberries are mildly sour. Adding sweet berries, creamy yogurt, and honey makes this smoothie extra delicious.

2 cups plain whole-milk yogurt

½ cup frozen blueberries

½ cup frozen chopped strawberries

1 cup Immune-Tune Astragalus Infusion (page 45) or lemonade

1 ounce Elderberry Antiviral Syrup (page 49) or store-bought syrup

1 tablespoon astragalus root powder

1 tablespoon rose hip powder

1 to 2 tablespoons honey or maple syrup (optional)

1. Put the yogurt, blueberries, strawberries, astragalus infusion, elderberry syrup, astragalus powder, rose hip powder, and honey, if desired, in a blender. Blend until smooth.

2. Pour the smoothie into a clean 32-ounce mason jar or glass and enjoy. Cover any remaining smoothie with a tight lid, and store in the refrigerator for up to 2 days.

NOTE: Do not use fresh or rehydrated elderberries in your smoothie. They can be emetic (make you throw up) when consumed this way. You can adjust the consistency of the smoothie to your liking by adding either more juice/infusion or yogurt. If you do not have the herbal powders, you can leave them out and the smoothie will still be beneficial to your health.

Goldenrod Decongestant Tisane

MAKES: 4 cups

This tisane helps clear congestion from the sinuses and lungs during and after infections. Goldenrod is rich in tannins that tighten mucous membranes and make the tisane taste like black tea. Depending on the severity of the congestion and how much tisane you drink, it can be 1 to 3 days before the benefits take full effect.

¼ cup fresh goldenrod
  leaves and flowers
  or 4 teaspoons dried,
  cut, and sifted

4 cups boiling water
Honey, for serving
  (optional)

1. Put the goldenrod in a large teapot, then cover with the boiling water. Cover with a lid and steep for 20 to 60 minutes, depending on how strong you like the tisane to taste.

2. Pour the tisane through a tea strainer into a clean 32-ounce mason jar.

3. Sweeten with honey to taste, if desired. Enjoy the tisane straight from the jar, or pour into a mug to drink. Store any remaining tisane in a covered jar in the refrigerator for up to 3 days.

NOTE: Drink 4 cups of tisane a day until congestion is relieved. Sometimes drinking too much goldenrod tisane can dry the sinus mucous membranes too much. If this is the case, you can switch to Throat-Soothing Linden Infusion (page 54) to soothe the mucous membranes of the sinuses.

Throat-Soothing Linden Infusion

MAKES: 4 cups

Linden soothes irritated, inflamed, and swollen mucous membranes of the entire throat, tonsils, and esophagus. Linden can be prepared as a tisane or an infusion. Linden tisane is a classic French cold and flu remedy. Linden infusion tastes floral and sweet. The infusion extracts more of the mucilaginous constituents of the plant and so is better for sore throats than the tisane. It can be enjoyed ice cold or warm with honey, which is also soothing and hydrating to the throat.

1 ounce dried whole linden flowers or ½ ounce dried, cut, and sifted

4 cups boiling water
Honey, for serving (optional)

1. Put the linden flowers in a 32-ounce mason jar, then fill the jar to the top with the boiling water. Cover with a tight lid, and steep for a minimum of 4 hours or up to overnight.

2. Line the mouth of a ceramic drip coffee filter with a straining cloth. Pour the infusion through the filter into a clean 32-ounce mason jar.

3. Gather the corners of the straining cloth, and wring the cloth to squeeze as much liquid from the flowers as you can.

4. Sweeten with honey to taste, if desired. Enjoy the infusion straight from the jar, or pour into a mug to drink. Store any remaining infusion in a covered jar in the refrigerator for up to 2 days.

NOTE: Enjoy this infusion frequently until symptoms subside. You can drink it cool over ice, which makes it more viscous and feels soothing on an inflamed throat and tonsils. Or you can drink it warm so that it is not as thick, which some folks prefer. If this recipe tastes too strong, make it with ½ ounce of whole blossoms.

Warm-the-Chills Spice Decoction

MAKES: 4 cups

A mug of warm spiced tea will enhance circulation and warm you from head to toe when you have the chills or a fever that makes you feel cold. The spices in this recipe are all antimicrobial, helping you fight infections. You can decoct these mulling spices in water, cider, or wine. When blending the spices, make extra and store them in an airtight container to use for spiced tea.

1 teaspoon cinnamon chips or ½ cinnamon stick

½ teaspoon dried ginger root

1 teaspoon cardamom seeds, removed from whole pods

½ teaspoon whole cloves

1 teaspoon fennel seeds

5 cups water, cider, milk, or red wine

Honey, for serving (optional)

Cream, for serving (optional)

1. In a saucepot or small soup pot, combine the cinnamon, ginger, cardamom, cloves, and fennel seeds. Cover with the water. Bring to a boil.

2. Reduce the heat to a simmer. Simmer for 20 to 40 minutes. Remove from the heat.

3. Pour the decoction through a tea strainer into a clean 32-ounce mason jar.

4. Add honey and cream to taste, if desired. Enjoy the decoction straight from the jar, or pour into a mug to drink. Store any remaining decoction in a covered jar in the refrigerator for up to 4 days.

NOTE: Avoid adding black pepper or hot pepper to your spice blend because they drive up inflammation in the body. Add sliced apples to the pot as it simmers for a sweet, fruity flavor.

Lymph-Mover Cleavers Infusion

MAKES: 4 cups

Cleavers is a popular herb in various parts of the world, its use dating back as far as ancient Greece and traditional Chinese medicine. This simple infusion supports the lymphatic system's ability to carry immune cells around the body and transport dead pathogens and their by-products to the pathways of elimination.

1 ounce dried cleavers   **4 cups boiling water**

1. Put the cleavers in a 32-ounce mason jar, then fill the jar to the top with the boiling water. Cover with a tight lid, and steep for a minimum of 4 hours or up to overnight.

2. Line the mouth of a ceramic drip coffee filter with a straining cloth. Pour the infusion through the filter into a clean 32-ounce mason jar.

3. Gather the corners of the straining cloth, and wring the cloth to squeeze as much liquid from the herbs as you can.

4. Enjoy the infusion straight from the jar, or pour into a mug to drink. Store any remaining infusion in a covered jar in the refrigerator for up to 2 days.

NOTE: For a more varied infusion, make it with a trio of immune-boosting herbs: ⅓ ounce of dried cleavers, ⅓ ounce of dried red clover blossoms, and ⅓ ounce of dried astragalus root.

Mullein Milk Lung Healer

MAKES: 4 cups

Mullein leaves heal lungs that are troubled with bronchitis, asthma, and chronic coughs. Traditionally, the leaves are brewed with milk and sweetened with honey to support lung health. Adding cinnamon or Warm-the-Chills Spice Decoction (page 55) makes the drink extra tasty and breaks up congestion.

½ ounce dried, cut, and sifted mullein leaves

2 cups boiling water

2 teaspoons cinnamon chips or 1 cinnamon stick

2 cups whole milk

1 teaspoon honey

1. Put the dried mullein leaves in a 16-ounce mason jar, then fill the jar to the top with the boiling water. Cover with a tight lid, and steep for a minimum of 4 hours or up to overnight.

2. Line the mouth of a ceramic drip coffee filter with a straining cloth. Pour the infusion through the filter into a clean 32-ounce mason jar.

3. Gather the corners of the straining cloth, and wring the cloth to squeeze as much liquid from the mullein as you can.

4. Pour the mullein infusion into a saucepot, and add the cinnamon chips. Cover and simmer for 10 minutes. Remove from the heat.

5. Pour the infusion through a tea strainer into a clean 32-ounce mason jar.

6. Add the milk, and stir in the honey. Enjoy the infusion straight from the jar throughout the day, or pour into a mug to drink. Store any remaining infusion in a covered jar in the refrigerator for up to 4 days.

NOTE: Mullein leaves have small hairs that can be irritating to the throat. Make sure to use a straining cloth with a weave tight enough to trap the hairs. Cheesecloth has too loose a weave.

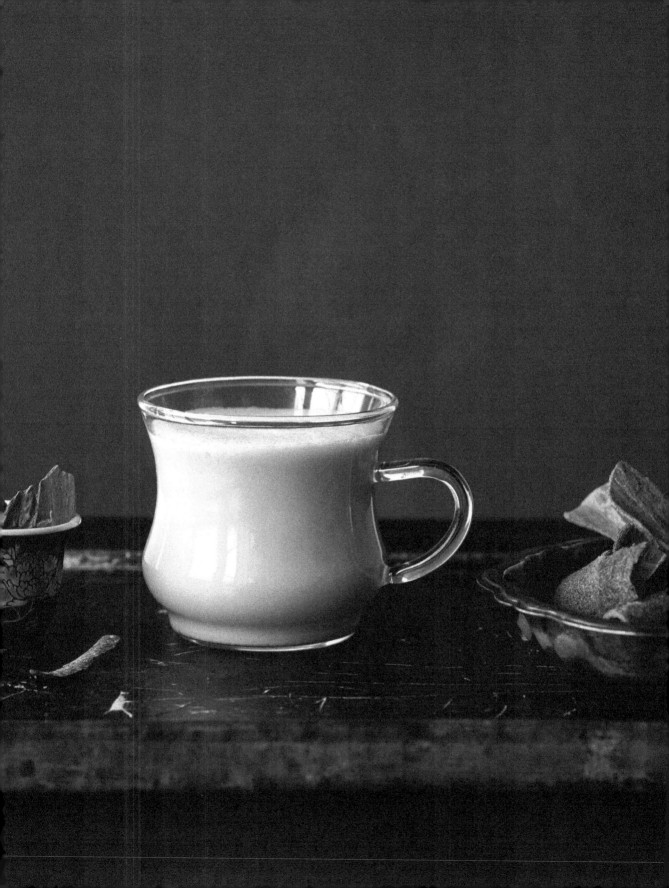

CHAPTER 5

For the Digestive System

Digestion is often considered the seat of health. Through the digestive system, the body obtains the necessary nutrients for the organs to function. The colon is an ecosystem teeming with beneficial microscopic life that assimilates nutrients. It provides hormones and mood-enhancing chemicals, such as serotonin and dopamine. Many organs are involved with the digestive process, including the liver, stomach, gallbladder, pancreas, and intestines. When any of these are injured, inflamed, or diseased, health suffers in noticeable ways.

This chapter showcases the most effective herbs to help your digestive system operate at its best. It includes so-called bitter herbs, which are known to support digestion, metabolism, elimination, and liver function. You'll also find mucilaginous herbs, which restore the integrity of the mucous membrane that lines the entire digestive tract. This lining is home to our microbiome and many immune cells. You will also find numerous recipes that include aromatic herbs, which kill pathogens and ease gut spasms.

The mixture of bitter, mucilaginous, and aromatic herbs in the recipes of this chapter will help promote overall digestive health and full-body well-being.

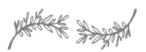

Mint and Chamomile Tisane to Ease the Belly

MAKES: 4 cups

Many people know mint and chamomile as calming teas for the mind, but they also offer digestive relief. In this tisane, they work in tandem to calm gut spasms, easing gas pains. They also subdue nausea, especially when the nausea is a symptom of anxiety and stress. You can use dried mint and chamomile, which are easy to find in grocery stores, or use fresh herbs that you can easily grow in patio pots or in a garden.

4 teaspoons dried, cut, and sifted mint leaves or ¼ cup fresh (any variety of mint that you enjoy works well, including peppermint, spearmint, apple mint, or chocolate mint)

4 teaspoons dried whole chamomile flowers or ¼ cup fresh

4 cups boiling water

1. Put the mint and chamomile in a teapot, then cover with the boiling water. Cover with a lid, and steep for 20 minutes.

2. Pour the tisane through a tea strainer into a clean 32-ounce mason jar. Enjoy straight from the jar, or pour into a mug to drink. Store any remaining tisane in a covered jar in the refrigerator for up to 3 days.

NOTE: You can add a tablespoon of Ginger Syrup to Ease an Upset Stomach (page 62) to ease your belly even more while also giving you some sweet spice.

Ginger Syrup to Ease an Upset Stomach

MAKES: 2 cups

Much loved for its sweet and spicy flavor, ginger is a superior herb when it comes to helping the digestive process. It quells an upset stomach, reduces cramps, relieves gas, and lessens stomach pain and bloating. Ginger also enhances blood circulation to the digestive tract, increasing nutrient absorption. This tasty syrup can be taken by the tablespoon on its own or stirred into tisane, bubbly water, or hot water with lemon. It can also be added to an after-dinner cocktail or hot toddy.

2 tablespoons chopped fresh ginger root or 1 tablespoon dried

2 cups water
1 cup honey or sugar

1. In a small saucepot, combine the ginger and water. Bring to a boil.

2. Reduce the heat to a simmer. Simmer until the water has reduced by half. Remove from the heat.

3. Line the mouth of a ceramic drip coffee filter with a straining cloth. Pour the decoction through the filter into a clean 16-ounce mason jar.

4. Gather the corners of the straining cloth, and wring the cloth to squeeze as much liquid from the ginger as you can.

5. Add the honey to the warm decoction. Stir until completely incorporated, creating a syrup. Cover the jar tightly, label, and store in the refrigerator for up to 6 months.

NOTE: Using dried ginger will make this syrup hotter and spicier than if you use fresh. You can create your own ginger ale by stirring a tablespoon of syrup into a glass of bubbly water.

Ginger-Blueberry Shrub for Better Digestion

MAKES: 2 cups

An herbal shrub is a drink made from vinegar, fruit, and a sweetener such as sugar or honey. This fun and tasty shrub brings together the digestive benefits of ginger, blueberries, and apple cider vinegar. You can add a spoonful of this remedy to bubbly water, warm water with lemon, and cocktails.

1½ cups apple cider vinegar

1 cup chopped fresh ginger root or ½ cup dried

1 cup frozen blueberries
½ cup honey

1. To pasteurize the vinegar, pour it into a nonmetal (Pyrex or ceramic-lined) pot and bring to a boil. Remove from the heat. Let cool to room temperature.

2. Put the ginger and blueberries in a 16-ounce mason jar, then cover with the vinegar.

3. Stir in the honey. Cover the jar with a tight lid. If using a metal lid, lay a square of unbleached wax paper between the lid and the vinegar. For long-term storage of vinegar, use a plastic food-safe lid. Label the jar, and let infuse for 6 weeks away from direct sunlight.

4. Line the mouth of a ceramic drip coffee filter with a straining cloth. Pour the shrub through the filter into a 2-cup measuring cup with a spout.

5. Gather the corners of the straining cloth, and wring the cloth to squeeze as much liquid from the plant material as you can.

6. Pour the shrub through a small funnel into 2 clean (8-ounce) Boston round amber bottles. Cover with tight plastic lids and label. Shrubs can be stored for up to 1 year when using pasteurized vinegar. Refrigeration will extend the shelf life as well.

NOTE: Be sure to put the vinegar in the jar before the honey so that you can combine them more easily.

After-Dinner Ginger and Mint Tisane

MAKES: 4 cups

If you're feeling bloated or overly full after a big meal or if you simply want some digestive relief, try this tisane. It brings together the medicinal benefits of ginger and mint in a delicious, stomach-soothing beverage that combines the methods of making a decoction and a tisane.

2 teaspoons dried ginger root or 2 tablespoons chopped fresh

5 cups water
4 teaspoons dried mint leaves or ¼ cup fresh

Honey or Ginger Syrup to Ease an Upset Stomach (page 62), for serving

1. In a saucepot, combine the ginger and water. Bring to a boil.

2. Reduce the heat to a simmer. Simmer for 40 minutes, or until the liquid has reduced to 4 cups. Remove from the heat.

3. Add the mint leaves, cover the pot, and let infuse for 20 minutes.

4. Pour the tisane through a tea strainer into a clean 32-ounce mason jar.

5. Stir in honey to taste. Enjoy the tisane straight from the jar, or pour into a mug to drink. Store any remaining tisane in a covered jar in the refrigerator for up to 4 days.

NOTE: This tisane is a refreshing palate cleanser on those evenings when you are too full for dessert but still want a tasty treat.

Aromatic Seed Tisane to Relieve Gas Pain

MAKES: 4 cups

You may already use aromatic seeds when cooking meals, but you may not be aware that they can be steeped in hot water to help relieve gas cramping, pain, and bloating in the intestines. Their antispasmodic aromatic oils ease cramps and release the buildup of gas. If you are short on any of the ingredients, you can substitute parsley, dill, or cumin seeds for them in the same ratio.

1 tablespoon fennel seeds

1 tablespoon coriander seeds

1 tablespoon celery seeds

1 tablespoon cardamom pods, crushed

4 cups water

1. In a saucepot, combine the fennel seeds, coriander seeds, celery seeds, cardamom, and water. (The seeds may be crushed with a mortar and pestle first to release their aromatic oils, if you like.) Cover, bring to a boil, then immediately reduce the heat to low. Simmer for 5 minutes. Remove from the heat. Steep for 20 minutes.

2. Pour the tisane through a tea strainer into a clean 32-ounce mason jar. Enjoy straight from the jar, or pour into a mug to drink. Store any remaining tisane in a covered jar in the refrigerator for up to 4 days.

NOTE: The tisane can also be made by combining all the ingredients in a large mason jar with boiling water and letting it steep for 20 minutes. You can then pour it through a strainer or leave it as is. The seeds will sink to the bottom of the jar, and you can drink the tisane off the top. You can chew on the soaked seeds if you enjoy their flavor (just avoid the cardamom pods). If digestive upset is a chronic issue that bothers you, carry this tisane with you, keeping it warm in a thermos, and sip throughout the day.

Premeal Dandelion, Orange, and Fennel Bitters

MAKES: 2 cups

Taking a teaspoonful of these digestive bitters at the start of a meal will get your entire digestive system ready to work. Used across Europe for centuries, bitters help stimulate the bitter receptors on the tongue, increase saliva production, and promote digestive juices such as stomach acid, bile, and enzymes to better break down your food. If you find the flavor of bitters too strong, you can add a teaspoon to a sweet mocktail or cocktail to dilute the taste.

1 cup chopped fresh dandelion root or ½ cup dried

½ cup chopped organic orange peel, including the white pith

¼ cup crushed fennel seeds

2 cups 100-proof vodka

1. In a clean 16-ounce mason jar, combine the dandelion root, orange peel, fennel seeds, and vodka. Cover with a tight lid, label, and let infuse for 6 weeks away from direct sunlight.

2. Line the mouth of a ceramic drip coffee filter with a straining cloth. Pour the bitters through the filter into a clean 2-cup measuring cup with a spout.

3. Pour the bitters through a small funnel into 2 clean (8-ounce) Boston round amber bottles. Cover with tight lids and label. Take a teaspoonful 15 minutes before a meal. Tinctures keep indefinitely due to their alcohol content.

NOTE: You can also take these bitters after a meal to help aid digestion after eating. Dandelion can be harvested ("weeded") any time the ground is not frozen. In spring and fall, the roots will be larger and sweeter; in the middle of the growing season, the roots will be smaller and more bitter. Only dig up the root after identifying the plant with 100 percent certainty and from unpolluted land. Rinse the root, pat it dry, and chop into small pieces.

Soothing Tisane with Lemon Balm and Catnip

MAKES: 4 cups

This bright and fragrant tisane is simple to make but goes a long way toward soothing your digestive system. The pairing of lemon balm and catnip helps ease abdominal pain, cramps, discomfort, and gas. The herbs also double as anxiety relief, helping quell butterflies in the belly and promote an overall sense of calm.

2 tablespoons fresh catnip or 2 teaspoons dried

2 tablespoons fresh lemon balm or 2 teaspoons dried

4 cups boiling water
Honey, for serving (optional)

1. Put the catnip and lemon balm in a teapot, then cover with the boiling water. Cover with a lid, and steep for 20 minutes.

2. Pour the tisane through a tea strainer into a clean 32-ounce mason jar.

3. Stir in honey to taste, if desired. Enjoy the tisane straight from the jar, or pour into a mug to drink. Store any remaining tisane in a covered jar in the refrigerator for up to 4 days.

NOTE: This tisane can be made stronger by adding more herb, and it can be sweetened with honey or Ginger Syrup to Ease an Upset Stomach (see page 62).

Burdock Root Chai for a Healthy Gut

MAKES: 4 cups

Burdock root is a digestive bitter that also provides food for the symbiotic gut microbes in the form of inulin. Adding this earthy root to the warming spices found in chai increases blood flow to the gut, supporting digestive function. Burdock root is rich in vitamins and minerals that nourish the whole body and its functions.

¼ cup chopped fresh burdock root or 2 tablespoons dried

1 teaspoon cinnamon chips or ½ cinnamon stick

½ teaspoon dried ginger

4 cardamom pods, crushed

4 whole cloves

1 teaspoon fennel seeds

5 cups water

1. In a saucepot, combine the burdock, cinnamon, ginger, cardamom, cloves, fennel seeds, and water. Bring to a boil.

2. Reduce the heat to a simmer. Partially cover the pot and simmer for 40 minutes, or until the liquid has reduced to about 4 cups. Remove from the heat.

3. Pour the chai through a tea strainer into a clean 32-ounce mason jar.

4. Enjoy straight from the jar, or pour into a mug to drink. Store any remaining chai in a covered jar in the refrigerator for up to 2 days.

NOTE: Burdock is a common weed. The root can be harvested, cleaned, chopped, and laid flat in a basket to dry. You can add a dash of honey or cream to this chai, if you wish.

Marshmallow Root Infusion to Coat the Digestive Tract

MAKES: 4 cups

You may know marshmallow as a fluffy white confection, but it is also the name of the plant the confection was originally made from. Marshmallow root's mucilaginous properties soothe and restore the necessary mucous membrane that lines the entire digestive tract. This infusion is especially helpful for people who have ulcers, inflamed bowels, colitis, or irritable bowel syndrome. The infusion can be consumed daily in whatever amount feels good to you until your symptoms resolve.

1 ounce dried
  marshmallow root
  or leaf

4 cups boiling water

1. Put the marshmallow root in a 32-ounce mason jar, then fill the jar to the top with the boiling water. Cover with a tight lid, and steep for a minimum of 4 hours or up to overnight.

2. Line the mouth of a ceramic drip coffee filter with a straining cloth. Pour the infusion through the filter into a clean 32-ounce mason jar.

3. Gather the corners of the straining cloth, and wring the cloth to squeeze as much liquid from the marshmallow root as you can.

4. Drink the infusion straight from the jar, pour into a glass over ice, or reheat by the mugful to enjoy warm. Store any remaining infusion in a covered jar in the refrigerator for up to 2 days.

NOTE: The mucilaginous components of marshmallow and all plants extract best in cool water. You can refrigerate the infusion for an hour before straining to increase the extraction. Dried marshmallow leaf can be substituted for the root in the same ratio.

Roasted Dandelion Root Decoction to Ease Heartburn

MAKES: 2 cups

This roasted dandelion root decoction is bitter, nutty, and slightly sweet. Dandelion root supports all aspects of digestion and elimination but is particularly effective at easing acid reflux. It may take a couple weeks of drinking this decoction before you notice a reduction in heartburn symptoms. Roasted dandelion root is similar in flavor to coffee and is often used as a caffeine-free substitute or is added to dilute coffee's uncomfortable side effects, which can include heartburn.

3 tablespoons roasted dandelion root

3 cups water

Cream, for serving (optional)

Honey or maple syrup, for serving (optional)

1. In a saucepot, combine the dandelion root and water. Bring to a boil.

2. Reduce the heat to a simmer. Simmer for 30 minutes, or until the liquid has reduced to about 2 cups. Remove from the heat.

3. Pour the decoction through a tea strainer into a mug to drink.

4. Stir in cream and honey to taste, if desired.

NOTE: Although you can purchase roasted dandelion root, you can also harvest your own. Harvest 6 tablespoons of root, wash, pat dry, and chop into small pieces. To roast, preheat the oven to 250°F, spread the pieces out on a baking sheet, and bake for 20 to 40 minutes, or until the roots are fully dry and slightly crunchy. They will have a toasted smell.

Warming Decoction for Liver and Gut Health

MAKES: 4 cups

This warming decoction brings together a trio of bitter roots, their flavors softened with the sweet anise taste of licorice and the bright spicy notes of ginger. Use this decoction when your digestion feels sluggish, you need extra liver support, or you have problems with chronic constipation.

2 teaspoons dried burdock root

1 teaspoon dried dandelion root

½ teaspoon dried yellow dock root

¼ teaspoon dried licorice root

¼ teaspoon dried ginger root

5 cups water

1. In a saucepot, combine the burdock, dandelion, yellow dock, licorice, ginger, and water. Bring to a boil.

2. Reduce the heat to low. Simmer for 40 minutes, or until the water has reduced to about 4 cups. Remove from the heat.

3. Pour the decoction through a tea strainer into a mug to drink.

4. Pour any remaining decoction through the strainer into a 32-ounce mason jar, cover, and store in the refrigerator for up to 4 days.

NOTE: You can enjoy a cup of this decoction before meals to support the liver and digestive function or in larger amounts throughout the day to relieve chronic constipation.

Mugwort, Fennel, and Chamomile Bedtime Bitters

MAKES: 1 cup

These bitters are a pleasant evening treat that will prepare you for sleep. The mugwort, fennel, and chamomile work together to ease any digestive upsets and calm the nervous system for a more restful night. You can add a teaspoon to a glass of bubbly water for an after-dinner drink or to a mug of warm water and honey before heading to bed. Alternatively, you can leave the bitters by the bed to take a sip from before going to sleep.

½ cup chopped fresh mugwort leaves or ¼ cup dried, cut, and sifted

2 tablespoons fennel seeds

¼ cup fresh chamomile flowers or 2 tablespoons dried

1 cup 100-proof vodka

1. Put the mugwort, fennel, and chamomile in an 8-ounce mason jar, then fill the jar to the top with the vodka, making sure the herbs are covered. Cover with a tight lid, label, and let infuse for 6 weeks away from direct sunlight.

2. Line the mouth of a ceramic drip coffee filter with a straining cloth. Pour the bitters through the filter into a clean 8-ounce mason jar.

3. Gather the corners of the straining cloth, and wring the cloth to squeeze as much liquid from the herbs as you can.

4. Pour the bitters through a small funnel into a clean (8-ounce) Boston round amber bottle. Cover with a tight lid and label. Tinctures keep indefinitely due to their alcohol content.

NOTE: You can make a tincture with any one of these herbs for a similar effect. If you have fresh plant material, fill the jar to the top with it. If you have dried plant material, fill the jar no more than halfway with plant material and then fill the jar to the top with 100-proof vodka.

Gut-Heal Tisane

MAKES: 4 cups

This tisane incorporates three herbs that ease digestive distress and irritation. Plantain leaf soothes and heals the lining of the gut. Calendula supports digestive function, relieving inflammation and irritation. Cinnamon adds a nice flavor to the tisane, soothes the lining of the gut, and relieves cramping.

¼ cup dried plantain leaf

¼ cup dried calendula flowers

4 teaspoons cinnamon chips or 1 cinnamon stick

4 cups boiling water

Honey, for serving (optional)

1. Put the plantain leaf, calendula, and cinnamon in a teapot, then cover with the boiling water. Cover with a lid, and steep for 20 minutes.

2. Pour the tisane through a tea strainer into a clean 32-ounce mason jar.

3. Sweeten with honey to taste, if desired. Enjoy the tisane straight from the jar, or pour into a mug to drink. Store any remaining tisane in a covered jar in the refrigerator for up to 2 days.

NOTE: Plantain leaf (*Plantago major* or *Plantago lanceolata*) is a very common weed that loves to grow around humans. There are no dangerous look-alikes. If this is a plant that grows in your area, you will likely see it everywhere you go, including in driveways, in sidewalk cracks, and along walking paths.

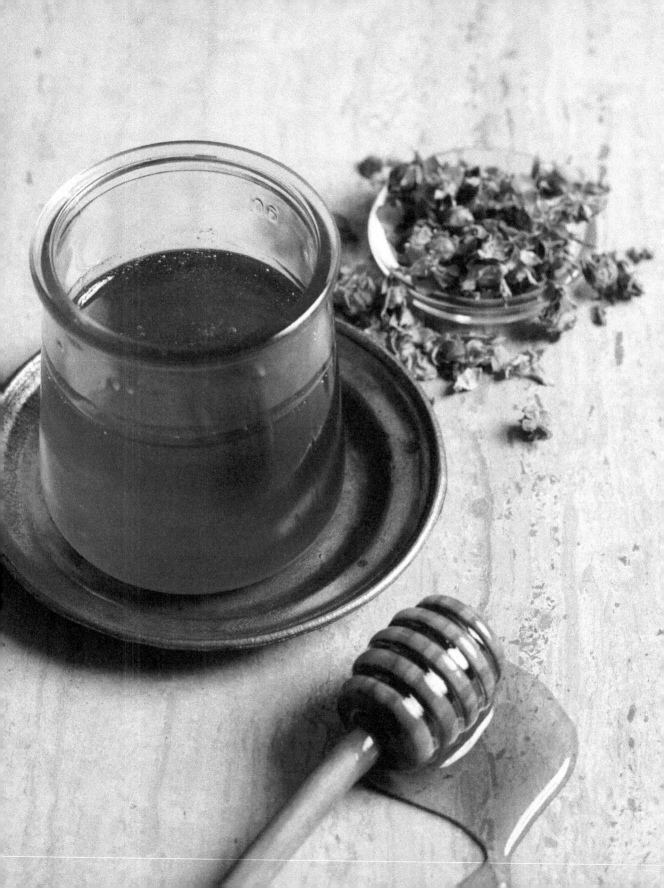

For Skin, Nails, and Hair

When it comes to promoting healthy skin, nails, and hair, many people think of topical balms, creams, and oils, but you can also support these parts of your body by drinking herbal infused drinks. This is because our internal health is often reflected in our outward appearance.

This chapter provides an array of infusions—from tisanes and decoctions to herb-infused vinegars and honey—that support internal health and fortify skin, hair, and nails. You'll find recipes that promote collagen production for elastic skin, that target inflamed or damaged skin, and that support bodily well-being for healthy cell growth. As a bonus, a few recipes can double as topical treatments for the skin.

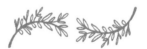

Multi-Herb Skin Tonic

MAKES: 4 cups

If you are looking for an all-round skin tonic, look no further than this nourishing four-herb infusion. The stinging nettle leaf and oat straw provide protein for healthy skin tissue, and the hawthorn flower and leaf promote collagen production. Rounding out the tonic is horsetail, an herb rich in silica, which helps keep skin elastic. If that wasn't enough, all of these herbs provide an array of minerals and vitamins that foster healthy skin, hair, and nails.

⅓ ounce dried stinging nettle leaf

⅓ ounce dried oat straw

⅓ ounce dried hawthorn flower and leaf

1 tablespoon dried horsetail herb

4 cups boiling water

1. Put the stinging nettle, oat straw, hawthorn, and horsetail in a 32-ounce mason jar, then fill the jar to the top with the boiling water. Stir the herbs to incorporate. Cover with a tight lid, and steep for a minimum of 4 hours or up to overnight.

2. Line the mouth of a ceramic drip coffee filter with a straining cloth. Pour the infusion through the filter into a clean 32-ounce mason jar.

3. Gather the corners of the straining cloth, and wring the cloth to squeeze as much liquid from the herbs as you can.

4. Enjoy the tonic straight from the jar, or pour into a glass over ice to drink. Store any remaining tonic in a covered jar in the refrigerator for up to 2 days.

NOTE: To improve the health and integrity of your hair, skin, and nails, drink this infusion at least once a week.

Soothing Skin Infusion with Comfrey, Mallow, and Rose

MAKES: 4 cups

This nourishing infusion is an ideal treatment for inflamed, irritated, or dry skin. It contains a mixture of herbs that help coat internal mucous membranes, soothe and protect skin tissue, and restore overall skin health. The healing mucilage components of these plants extract best in cold water, so after you have steeped the infusion, place it in the refrigerator to complete the process.

½ cup dried
  comfrey leaf
  (not root)

½ cup dried
  marshmallow leaf
¼ cup dried rose petals

Pinch dried tulsi
  (optional)
4 cups boiling water

1. Put the comfrey, marshmallow, rose petals, and tulsi, if desired (it adds flavor), in a 32-ounce mason jar, then fill the jar to the top with the boiling water. Stir the herbs to incorporate. Cover with a tight lid, and steep for a minimum of 3 hours. Once at room temperature, refrigerate for a minimum of 1 hour.

2. Line the mouth of a ceramic drip coffee filter with a straining cloth. Pour the infusion through the filter into a clean 32-ounce mason jar.

3. Gather the corners of the straining cloth, and wring the cloth to squeeze as much liquid from the herbs as you can.

4. Enjoy the infusion straight from the jar, or pour into a mug to drink. Store any remaining infusion in a covered jar in the refrigerator for up to 2 days.

NOTE: This infusion can be applied topically with a washcloth or added to bathwater. Only use dried comfrey leaf in this infusion rather than comfrey root, which is for external use only.

Antioxidant Infusion for Healthy Skin

MAKES: 4 cups

The pleasing combination of rose hips, green tea, and lemon balm in this infusion offers an abundance of nutrients and antioxidants that protect skin from premature aging. You can also apply this infusion topically to tone the skin and relieve inflammation.

¼ cup chopped dried
 rose hips
5 cups water

1 tablespoon dried
 green tea
2 tablespoons dried
 lemon balm

Honey, for serving
 (optional)

1. In a saucepot, combine the rose hips and water. Bring to a boil.

2. Reduce the heat to a simmer. Simmer for 40 minutes, or until the liquid has reduced to about 4 cups. Remove from the heat.

3. Add the green tea and lemon balm. Cover the pot with a lid, and steep for 20 minutes.

4. Line the mouth of a ceramic drip coffee filter with a straining cloth. Pour the infusion through the filter into a clean 32-ounce mason jar.

5. Gather the corners of the straining cloth, and wring the cloth to squeeze as much liquid from the herbs as you can.

6. Stir in honey to taste, if desired. Enjoy the infusion straight from the jar, or pour into a mug to drink. Store any remaining infusion in a covered jar in the refrigerator for up to 4 days.

NOTE: This infusion is also enjoyable poured over ice into a glass with a slice of lemon. If you are using fresh rose hips, be sure to strain them as described to remove the hairs that surround their seeds, which can irritate the throat. These hairs should already be removed if you are using store-bought rose hips.

Linden and Elderflower Anti-Inflammatory Tisane

MAKES: 4 cups

The blending of linden blossoms and elderflower in this tisane produces a delicately sweet and floral beverage rich in anti-inflammatory compounds. Anti-inflammatory herbs are helpful when skin is inflamed, red, and irritated—for example, in cases of eczema and acne. When hair follicles become inflamed, they become red and irritated, and that can result in hair loss. You can also apply this tisane as a facial toner to soothe your skin or scalp.

¼ cup dried, cut, and sifted linden blossoms or 1 cup dried whole

¼ cup dried elderflowers

4 cups boiling water

1. Put the linden blossoms and elderflowers in a teapot, then cover with the boiling water. Cover with a lid, and steep for 20 minutes.

2. Pour the tisane through a tea strainer into a clean 32-ounce mason jar.

3. Enjoy straight from the jar, or pour into a mug to drink. Store any remaining tisane in a covered jar in the refrigerator for up to 2 days.

NOTE: If the flavor of the tisane is too strong, you can dilute it with water or lemonade. It can also be sweetened with honey. In the warmer months, you can pour this drink into a glass over ice for a more refreshing drink when you feel overheated. To use on your skin, dampen a washcloth with the tisane and wipe or leave the cloth on the skin for 10 minutes. Reapply frequently.

Dandelion Vinegar for Skin and Hair Enrichment

MAKES: 2 cups

This vinegar features dandelion, a common weed in gardens and lawns across North America, identifiable by its yellow spring flowers and smooth, toothed stemless leaves. Dandelion offers a variety of minerals and vitamins that enrich hair and skin and improve nail strength. It also supports the liver, which is vital to skin health, helping keep your skin clear and healthy. Dandelions contain inulin, a white sediment that forms in the remedy. It looks odd at first, but the inulin is beneficial for the gut microbiome and helpful to leave in the remedy.

2 cups apple cider vinegar

1 large or 2 small whole dandelion plants, including the roots

1. To pasteurize the vinegar, pour it into a nonmetal (Pyrex or ceramic-lined) pot and bring to a boil. Remove from the heat. Let cool to room temperature.

2. Harvest 1 or 2 dandelion plants, including the root. Clean the root with water. The leaves can be rinsed, if they are dirty. Pat dry. Chop the entire plant.

3. Lightly pack the plant into a 16-ounce mason jar, then fill the jar with the vinegar, being sure to cover all the plant material. Cover with a tight lid. If using a metal lid, lay a square of unbleached wax paper between the lid and the vinegar. For long-term storage of vinegar, use a plastic food-safe lid. Label the jar, and let infuse for 6 weeks away from direct sunlight. Consume the vinegar by the spoonful, add it to drinks, or use it as a base for salad dressing.

NOTE: The vinegar-soaked greens and roots can be eaten and used as garnishes on salad or rice. Although there are no dangerous look-alikes of dandelion, it is recommended to use a plant identification book to help you identify it if you are unfamiliar with the plant. (See page 66 for details on harvesting dandelion.)

Liver-Loving Roots Decoction for Healthy Skin

MAKES: 4 cups

The state of the skin is often a window to the health of the liver. If the liver is struggling to keep the blood healthy and free of unnecessary hormones and metabolites, we can develop skin problems. When we support the health and functioning of our liver, we support the health of our skin. This is a slightly bitter decoction, so it includes cinnamon for a hint of spice and the option of adding licorice for extra sweetness. Bitter herbs are generally beneficial for improving liver and digestive functions.

4 teaspoons dried
dandelion root
4 teaspoons dried
burdock root

1 cinnamon stick
¼ teaspoon licorice root
(optional)
5 cups water

Honey, for serving
(optional)

1. In a saucepot, combine the dandelion, burdock, cinnamon, licorice, if desired, and water. Bring to a boil.

2. Reduce the heat to a simmer. Cover the pot and simmer for 30 minutes, or until the liquid has reduced to about 4 cups. Remove from the heat. Steep for 20 minutes.

3. Pour the decoction through a tea strainer into a clean 32-ounce mason jar.

4. Sweeten with a dash of honey, if desired. Enjoy the decoction straight from the jar, or pour into a mug to drink. Store any remaining decoction in a covered jar in the refrigerator for up to 2 days.

NOTE: You can drink 4 cups of this decoction per week or more if necessary. You may need to consume it on a regular basis for 2 to 3 months before you notice improvements of chronic skin problems. This decoction also aids digestion. You can add 1 teaspoon of dried ginger root or 1 tablespoon of fresh ginger root to the blend for more digestive support and to spice the drink up and change the flavor.

Burdock Infusion for Clearer Skin

MAKES: 4 cups

This burdock infusion can provide lasting results in clearing stubborn skin conditions. It takes some time to take effect, so it will need to be drunk regularly over the span of a few months before you see results. Give it time, have patience, and you will be rewarded. This infusion has a nutty, earthy, and slightly bitter flavor. If you want to change the flavor, combine it with apple cider, hot chocolate, or coffee.

1 ounce dried burdock root

4 cups boiling water

1. Put the burdock in a 32-ounce mason jar, then fill the jar to the top with the boiling water. Cover with a tight lid, and steep for a minimum of 4 hours or up to overnight.

2. Line the mouth of a ceramic drip coffee filter with a straining cloth. Pour the infusion through the filter into a clean 32-ounce mason jar.

3. Gather the corners of the straining cloth, and wring the cloth to squeeze as much liquid from the root as you can.

4. Enjoy the infusion straight from the jar throughout the day, or pour into a glass over ice. Store any remaining infusion in a covered jar in the refrigerator for up to 3 days.

NOTE: Drink at least 1 cup of the infusion per day over the course of a few months. Burdock root can cause loose stools, so if you experience this, reduce the amount you drink.

Burdock and Echinacea Tincture to Treat Acne and Eczema

MAKES: 2 cups

This combination of burdock and echinacea roots supports skin health in a variety of ways and is especially helpful for people troubled by chronic acne or eczema. Both roots are anti-inflammatory, reducing the red irritation acne and eczema cause. Burdock works by improving the pathways and organs of metabolism and elimination, such as the liver, digestive process, and the kidneys. Echinacea supports the immune response by helping fight any infection that may be present and by modulating the inflammatory response of the immune system. When the immune system and systems of metabolism and elimination are working well, skin becomes less troubled and inflamed.

¼ cup dried burdock root

¼ cup dried Echinacea angustifolia root

2 cups 100-proof vodka

1. Put the burdock and echinacea in a 16-ounce mason jar, then fill the jar with the vodka. Cover with a tight lid, label, and let infuse for 6 weeks away from direct sunlight.

2. Pour the tincture through a tea strainer into a clean measuring cup with a spout.

3. Pour the tincture through a small funnel into 2 clean (8-ounce) Boston round amber bottles. Cover with tight lids and label. Tinctures keep indefinitely due to their alcohol content.

NOTE: Add up to 1 tablespoon of this tincture to a cup of bubbly water to drink before meals. Start with a small dose of 1 teaspoon and work your way up to what works for you. You can also add tincture to a cup of warm water with honey and lemon.

Collagen-Building Hawthorn Infusion

MAKES: 4 cups

Hawthorn is known to support the growth of collagen, which keeps our skin and joints flexible and supple and protects them from accelerated aging. This infusion is floral yet astringent in taste, similar to Earl Grey tea. Astringent herbs tighten and tone mucous membranes, including the skin. Hawthorn flowers add a subtle sweet flavor, like how bergamot sweetens Earl Grey tea. Hawthorn leaf infusion tastes nice iced or warm with honey.

1 ounce dried hawthorn leaves and flowers

4 cups boiling water

Honey, for serving (optional)

1. Put the hawthorn in a 32-ounce mason jar, then fill the jar to the top with the boiling water. Cover with a tight lid, and steep for a minimum of 4 hours or up to overnight.

2. Line the mouth of a ceramic drip coffee filter with a straining cloth. Pour the infusion through the filter into a clean 32-ounce mason jar.

3. Gather the corners of the straining cloth, and wring the cloth to squeeze as much liquid from the herbs as you can.

4. Add honey to sweeten, if desired. Enjoy the infusion directly from the jar, or pour into a glass over ice. Store any remaining infusion in a covered jar in the refrigerator for up to 2 days.

NOTES: Drink at least 4 cups of this infusion per week to gain its full benefits. You can also change this recipe to contain ½ ounce of dried hawthorn berries and ½ ounce of dried hawthorn leaves and flowers. This will add anti-inflammatory bioflavonoids and a berry flavor that will soften the astringency of the leaf.

Comfrey Infusion for Cell Repair

MAKES: 4 cups

This comfrey leaf infusion contains large amounts of allantoin, which is important for healthy cell regeneration. It aids in healing wounds and injuries while also keeping skin strong, flexible, and supple. Comfrey leaf is loaded with an array of minerals that strengthen hair and nails. Nails that have ridges, peel, or are soft are a sign that the body needs more minerals in the diet. Comfrey leaf infusion is an easy way to get the necessary minerals in a readily assimilable form.

1 ounce dried
  comfrey leaf

Pinch mint (optional)
4 cups boiling water

1. Put the comfrey and mint, if desired, in a 32-ounce mason jar, then fill the jar to the top with the boiling water. Stir to combine. Cover with a tight lid, and steep for a minimum of 4 hours or up to overnight.

2. Line the mouth of a ceramic drip coffee filter with a straining cloth. Pour the infusion through the filter into a clean 32-ounce mason jar.

3. Gather the corners of the straining cloth, and wring the cloth to squeeze as much liquid from the herbs as you can.

4. Enjoy the infusion straight from the jar, or pour into a mug to drink. Store any remaining infusion in a covered jar in the refrigerator for up to 2 days.

NOTE: Comfrey leaf is also excellent to apply topically to heal wounds, burns, rashes, and inflammations. Wrap the leftover leaf from the infusion in the straining cloth, and apply it to your skin as a compress. Comfrey infusion can be applied topically with a washcloth or in a foot soak, sitz bath, or body bath.

Vitamin and Mineral Herbal Vinegar

MAKES: 2 cups

The making of this vinegar extracts numerous antioxidants, vitamins, and minerals from stinging nettle leaf, dandelion leaf, and rose hips. The minerals help build strong nails, shiny hair, and smooth skin. This nourishing vinegar can be used as a condiment for food, a sour and slightly bitter addition to drinks, or on its own by the spoonful. All of these herbs could be harvested from a garden or the wild and dried, or purchased already dried.

2 cups apple cider vinegar

¼ cup dried stinging nettle leaf

¼ cup dried dandelion leaf

½ cup dried rose hips

1. To pasteurize the vinegar, pour it into a nonmetal (Pyrex or ceramic-lined) pot and bring to a boil. Remove from the heat. Let cool to room temperature.

2. Put the stinging nettle, dandelion, and rose hips in a 16-ounce mason jar, then fill the jar to the top with the vinegar. Cover with a tight lid. If using a metal lid, lay a square of unbleached wax paper between the lid and the vinegar. For long-term storage of vinegar, use a plastic food-safe lid. Label the jar, and let infuse for 6 weeks away from direct sunlight.

3. Line the mouth of a ceramic drip coffee filter with a straining cloth. Pour the vinegar through the filter into a measuring cup with a spout.

4. Pour the vinegar through a small funnel into 2 clean (8-ounce) Boston round amber bottles with plastic lids. Serve the vinegar by the spoonful, in a cup of bubbly water, or in a warm mug of lemon water and honey. The pasteurized vinegar can be stored for up to 2 years.

NOTE: You can use fresh herbs for this recipe, if you wish to harvest the herbs from a garden or weed patch in the fall when rose hips are ripe. Just be sure to pick newly grown nettle leaves rather than leaves that have seed stalks attached to them. When you have gathered all the fresh herbs, chop enough to fill the 16-ounce mason jar lightly packed, cover them with the pasteurized vinegar, and infuse for 6 weeks away from direct sunlight.

Cooling Rose Petal Honey

MAKES: 2 cups

Not only is rose petal honey a pleasing addition to all manner of drinks, but it also possesses anti-inflammatory properties that ease all manner of skin inflammations when taken internally and applied externally. The rose petals are edible, so there's no need to remove them from the honey. Gently rub the honey on inflamed skin or minor burns to cool and heal, or apply it as a face mask. The honey brings moisture and plumps the skin, while the rose petals soften and soothe irritations.

2 cups chopped fresh rose petals

2 cups honey, plus more as needed

1. In a bowl, stir together the rose petals and honey until well incorporated.

2. Pour the mixture through a wide-mouth funnel into a clean 16-ounce mason jar. Make sure the rose petals are covered with honey and the jar is full. Top off the jar with a little more honey, as needed. Cover with a tight lid and label. Stir the honey into tea, cocktails, mocktails, or smoothies by the spoonful (or more, as desired).

NOTE: You can use any rose petals that have a nice scent. Do not use rose petals from a florist; they are almost always treated with pesticides. Rose petal honey can also be spread on toast or drizzled on ice cream or yogurt.

Anti-Inflammatory Chamomile-Rose Spritzer

MAKES: 4 cups

This fun and delicious beverage is anti-inflammatory for the skin. Chamomile and rose cool and soothe irritated, inflamed skin from the inside out. When we have chronically inflamed and irritated skin, it is easy for our emotions to mirror this, and vice versa. As a side benefit, these herbs also soothe irritated inflamed emotions. The heat of a summer day can aggravate both conditions, so enjoy this beverage with friends to cool the body, skin, and emotions.

1 tablespoon dried chamomile flowers

1 tablespoon Cooling Rose Petal Honey (page 88)

2 cups boiling water

Ice, for serving

2 cups bubbly water or prosecco

Rose petals, for garnish (optional)

1. Put the chamomile flowers and rose honey in a teapot, then cover with the boiling water. Cover with a lid, and steep for 20 minutes.

2. Pour the tisane through a tea strainer into a clean 32-ounce mason jar. Once the tisane is at room temperature, add ice and the bubbly water.

3. Pour the tisane into wine or Champagne glasses.

4. Garnish each glass with a rose petal, if desired, and enjoy.

NOTE: You can make a chamomile tisane sweetened with rose honey and drink it warm to gain the same benefits. Steep 2 teaspoons of chamomile in 2 cups of boiling water. Strain through a tea strainer over a mug, and add 1 teaspoon of rose honey.

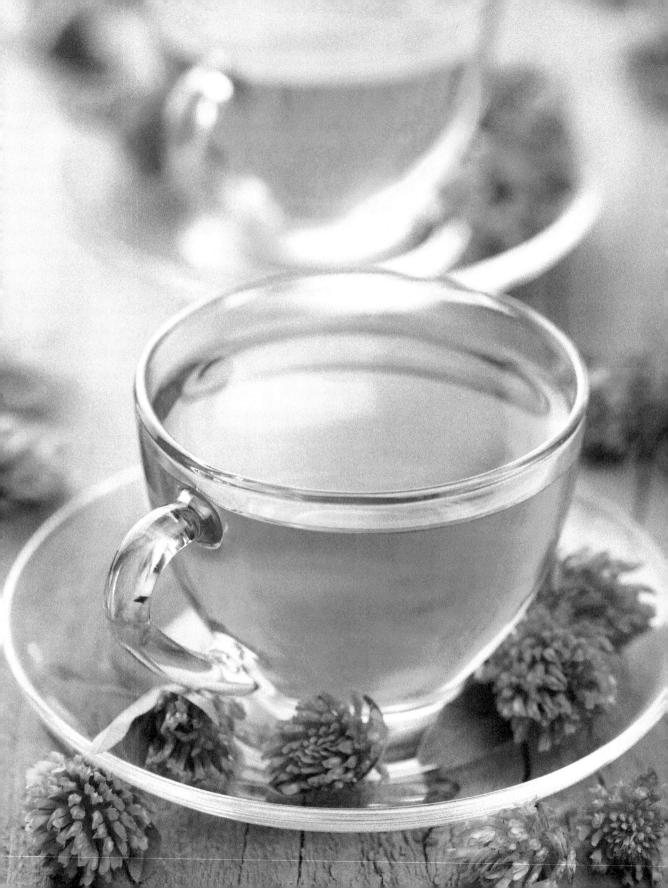

For the Reproductive System and Women's Health

Herbal medicine has been used across millennia to support female health and improve common women's health concerns. These recipes bring together some of the best herbs to promote well-being and ease discomfort for women at various stages of their life: while menstruating, during pregnancy, in postpartum recovery, and through menopause. Herbalism helps us understand that these natural stages of a woman's life are not problems that need "fixing" but are natural processes that benefit from care and nourishment.

The recipes in this chapter focus on different aspects of the reproductive system and women's health, sometimes to help with specific conditions or stages in life. If you are looking for other herbs to build health and resiliency through menstruation, pregnancy, nursing, motherhood, and menopause, chapter 11 offers an array of beneficial infusions. In particular, I prefer the Rotation of Herbal Infusions for Resiliency (page 155), a cornerstone self-care practice that could just as easily begin this chapter.

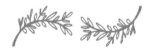

Rose Petal Elixir for Reproductive Health

MAKES: 2 cups

Rose is known to relieve a broad range of female reproductive system complaints that are connected to hormone fluctuations, easing the life transitions of puberty and menopause and increasing sexual vitality. This elixir can be taken by the dropperful, spoonful, in rose or other tisanes, or in bubbly water.

2 cups fresh rose petals, chopped, or 1 cup dried rose petals

1½ cups 100-proof vodka

½ cup Cooling Rose Petal Honey (page 88) or plain honey

1. Put the rose petals in a clean 16-ounce mason jar, then pour in the vodka.

2. Add the honey and stir. Cover the jar with a tight lid, label, and let infuse for 6 weeks away from direct sunlight.

3. Line the mouth of a ceramic drip coffee filter with a straining cloth. Pour the elixir through the filter into a clean 16-ounce mason jar.

4. Gather the corners of the straining cloth, and wring the cloth to squeeze as much liquid from the rose petals as you can.

5. Pour the elixir through a small funnel into 2 clean (8-ounce) Boston round amber bottles. Cover with tight lids and label. Elixirs store indefinitely due to their alcohol content.

NOTE: Any type of scented rose petals can be used. However, do not use roses from florists since they are usually sprayed with pesticides. Dried rose petals may be used in half the amount as fresh petals. Due to its alcohol content, this elixir should be avoided by pregnant or breastfeeding women.

Fertile Ground Red Clover Infusion

MAKES: 4 cups

The red clover in this infusion offers minerals, vitamins, and hormonal precursors that increase fertility. The red raspberry leaf is considered a tonic for the uterus, enhancing its ability to grow a new life. This infusion has an astringent yet floral taste. It can be enjoyed warm with honey to cut the astringency, if necessary.

1 ounce dried red clover blossoms

¼ cup dried red raspberry leaves

4 cups boiling water

Honey, for serving (optional)

1. Put the red clover blossoms and raspberry leaves in a 32-ounce mason jar, then fill the jar to the top with the boiling water. Cover with a tight lid, and steep for a minimum of 4 hours or up to overnight.

2. Line the mouth of a ceramic drip coffee filter with a straining cloth. Pour the infusion through the filter into a clean 32-ounce mason jar.

3. Gather the corners of the straining cloth, and wring the cloth to squeeze as much liquid from the herbs as you can.

4. Sweeten with a dash of honey, if desired. Enjoy the infusion straight from the jar, or pour into a mug to drink. Store any remaining infusion in a covered jar in the refrigerator for up to 2 days.

NOTE: You can drink up to 4 cups of this recipe per week. Make sure to use the whole red clover blossoms and not the leaves. The leaves are more likely to cause unwanted side effects or interactions with blood-thinning medications.

Mamma's Milk Nursing Tisane

MAKES: 4 cups

Fenugreek seeds and fennel seeds are common in kitchen pantries for cooking, but they are prized by herbalists as galactagogues, which are herbs that increase milk flow while nursing. This tisane is easy to make and can be enjoyed throughout the day.

4 teaspoons fenugreek seeds

4 teaspoons fennel seeds

4 cups boiling water

1. Put the fenugreek and fennel seeds in a teapot, then cover with the boiling water. Cover with a lid, and steep for 20 minutes.

2. Pour the tisane through a tea strainer into a clean 32-ounce mason jar. Enjoy straight from the jar, or pour into a mug to drink. Store any remaining tisane in a covered jar in the refrigerator for up to 3 days.

NOTE: In a rush? Rather than straining the herbs, you can simply put all the ingredients in a 32-ounce mason jar, allow it to steep for 20 minutes, then sip on the tisane throughout the day without straining. The seeds will sink to the bottom of the jar, but they can be chewed, if you like. If the tisane becomes too strong, you can strain the seeds out.

Fennel and Catnip Tisane for Colic Relief

MAKES: 4 cups

This tea helps ease baby colic, especially when the colic is a symptom of digestive distress or emotional unease. Fennel and catnip are specific for relieving gas pains and indigestion. Catnip is also known to calm and center babies' and children's minds and emotional states. When the mother drinks it, the baby gets the benefits through the breast milk. The tisane has a mildly sweet mint flavor with fennel- or licorice-flavor undertones.

4 teaspoons dried fennel seeds

4 teaspoons dried catnip leaf

4 cups boiling water

1. Put the fennel and catnip in a 32-ounce mason jar, then fill the jar to the top with the boiling water. Cover with a tight lid, and steep for 20 minutes.

2. Pour the tisane through a tea strainer into a clean 32-ounce mason jar. Enjoy straight from the jar, or pour into a mug to drink. Store any remaining tisane in a covered jar in the refrigerator for up to 2 days.

NOTE: Catnip tisane is also calming to help with sleep and can help lower a fever. Both are helpful properties for babies and can be relayed via the mother's milk.

Calming Postpartum Tisane

MAKES: 4 cups

As a new mother, it's easy to feel overwhelmed, stressed, and anxious. This delicious combination of lemon balm, rose petals, and oat tops calms the nerves and eases stress and anxiety without being overly sedating. Enjoy warm or over ice.

2 teaspoons dried lemon balm leaf

4 teaspoons dried rose petals

2 tablespoons dried oat tops

4 cups boiling water

1. Put the lemon balm, rose petals, and oat tops in a 32-ounce mason jar, then fill the jar to the top with the boiling water. Cover with a tight lid, and steep for 20 minutes.

2. Pour the tisane through a tea strainer into a clean 32-ounce mason jar. Enjoy straight from the jar, or pour into a mug to drink. Store any remaining tisane in a covered jar in the refrigerator for up to 2 days.

NOTE: Drink this tisane throughout the day or when you are feeling especially in need of a calming treat. This herb combination could be made into an elixir: Fill a jar half full with dried herbs or completely full with fresh herbs. Add 100-proof vodka to fill two-thirds of the jar. Fill the remaining one-third with honey.

Astragalus and Rose Hip Decoction for Women's Immunity

MAKES: 4 cups

This decoction is tailored to support immune health during pregnancy and afterward in postpartum recovery. Astragalus is a tough, woody root long used in traditional Chinese medicine for immune support. Rose hips are the fruit of the rose bush and are rich in nutrients, antioxidants, and immune-promoting properties. When decocted, they yield a pleasingly mild and sweet flavor.

¼ cup dried astragalus root

¼ cup dried rose hips

5 cups water

1. In a saucepot, combine the astragalus, rose hips, and water. Bring to a boil.

2. Reduce the heat to a simmer. Cover the pot and simmer for 30 minutes, or until the liquid has reduced to 4 cups. Remove from the heat. Steep for 20 minutes.

3. Pour the decoction through a tea strainer into a clean 32-ounce mason jar. Enjoy straight from the jar, or pour into a mug to drink. Store any remaining decoction in a covered jar in the refrigerator for up to 4 days.

NOTE: Both astragalus root and rose hips can be purchased in powdered form and added to yogurt and smoothies. Use 1 tablespoon of each per serving.

Ginger Tisane for Relief from Nausea and Cramps

MAKES: 4 cups

This ginger tisane is especially helpful in relieving nausea during pregnancy and also menstrual cramps. Fresh ginger root is preferred because it is not as spicy as dried ginger. As a bonus, this tisane can also help prevent motion sickness.

4 teaspoons grated
  fresh ginger root

4 cups boiling water

1. Put the ginger in a teapot, then cover with the boiling water. Cover with a lid, and steep for 20 minutes (or longer for a stronger flavor).

2. Pour the tisane through a tea strainer into a clean 32-ounce mason jar. Enjoy straight from the jar, or pour into a mug to drink. Store any remaining tisane in a covered jar in the refrigerator for up to 4 days.

NOTE: Because of its warming qualities, ginger is an excellent herb for folks who tend to run cold. This tisane tastes great with a dash of honey and a squeeze of lemon juice.

Women's Motherwort Elixir

MAKES: 2 cups

This motherwort elixir helps ease menstrual cramps and support heart health through menopause and beyond. Motherwort is native to Europe and Asia, though it has naturalized in many places in the world.

2 cups chopped fresh
 motherwort, flowering
 top of the plant

1½ cups 100-proof
 vodka
½ cup honey

1. Put the motherwort in a clean 16-ounce mason jar, then pour in the vodka.

2. Add the honey and stir. Cover the jar with a tight lid, label, and let infuse for 6 weeks away from direct sunlight.

3. Line the mouth of a ceramic drip coffee filter with a straining cloth. Pour the infusion through the filter into a clean 16-ounce mason jar.

4. Gather the corners of the straining cloth, and wring the cloth to squeeze as much liquid from the motherwort as you can. Be careful of the sharp plant parts that surround the flowers.

5. Pour the elixir through a small funnel into 2 clean (8-ounce) Boston round amber bottles. Cover with tight lids and label. Enjoy by the dropperful, by the spoonful, or mixed in bubbly water. Elixirs keep indefinitely due to their alcohol content.

NOTE: Motherwort (*Leonurus cardiaca*) is a weedy mint-family plant that spreads lots of seeds and grows well in a big pot. If you can harvest fresh flowering tops or find tincture made with fresh flowering tops, it is best. If all you have access to is dried motherwort, you only need to use 1 cup for this recipe.

Schisandra and Rose Vitality Smoothie

MAKES: 4 cups

This is a sweet-tart smoothie that provides full-body health by increasing stamina, energy, and sexual vitality. Schisandra is an adaptogen that supports the adrenal glands' ability to increase stamina and energy. It has also long been known as an herb that enhances sexual vitality in both men and women. Rose is an herb commonly associated with romance and love, not only due to its beauty and scent but also due to its aphrodisiac properties. Rose hips are full of nutrients that revitalize the whole body and improve blood circulation throughout.

1 teaspoon schisandra berry powder

1 tablespoon rose hip powder

1 tablespoon Cooling Rose Petal Honey (page 88) or plain honey

1 cup frozen strawberries, chopped

2 cups whole-milk plain yogurt, plus more as needed

1 cup lemonade or Calming Oat Straw Infusion (page 123), plus more as needed

1. Put the schisandra powder, rose hip powder, honey, strawberries, yogurt, and lemonade in a blender. Blend until smooth.

2. Add more lemonade to make the smoothie thinner or more yogurt to make it thicker, as desired.

3. Pour the smoothie into a glass. Store any remaining smoothie in a covered jar in the refrigerator for up to 2 days.

NOTE: Schisandra has a strong flavor, so if you find it too intense, you can reduce the amount in this recipe as you wish.

Cardamom-Rose Hot Chocolate

MAKES: 2 cups

This recipe adds an herbal twist to hot chocolate with cardamom and rose petals. It is a comforting treat, especially for pregnant, premenstrual, and menstruating women, and will help satiate any chocolate cravings. Rose petals are a supportive tonic for the entire reproductive system in all of its life stages. This delightful combination of herbs calms and awakens the mind with a feel-good vitality.

2 cups milk or milk substitute

6 whole cardamom pods, crushed

6 tablespoons dried rose petals

¼ cup cocoa powder

⅛ cup chocolate chips

¼ cup sugar or 2 tablespoons Cooling Rose Petal Honey (page 88)

1. In a small saucepot, combine the milk, cardamom, and rose petals. Bring to a simmer. Remove from the heat. Cover with a lid. Steep for 20 minutes.

2. Pour the infused milk through a tea strainer into a clean measuring cup with a spout, then return to the pot.

3. Add the cocoa powder, chocolate chips, and sugar. Whisk together while warming the infusion over medium-low heat until the chocolate and sugar have melted and fully incorporated with the milk. Remove from the heat.

4. Pour the hot chocolate into a large mug and enjoy.

NOTE: Adding a drop or two of rose water or ¼ teaspoon of vanilla extract can add more flavor. Depending on how bitter your cocoa powder is, you may want to add more sweetener.

Sage Infusions to Cool Night Sweats

MAKES: 1 cup honey; 2 cups tisane

Sage is a helpful herb for when women enter menopause. It can reduce the severity of hot flashes and night sweats. It can also ease other menopausal symptoms, such as panic, fatigue, and mental fog. Enjoy this sweet and savory tea during the day or after dinner. It makes for a lovely beverage and prepares you for heated nights.

FOR THE SAGE HONEY

1 cup finely chopped
  fresh sage leaves

1 cup honey

FOR THE TISANE

1 teaspoon sage honey

2 cups boiling water

TO MAKE THE SAGE HONEY

1. Put the sage and honey in a 16-ounce mason jar. Make sure the plant material is fully covered by the honey. Cover with a tight lid, label, and let infuse for 4 weeks away from direct sunlight.

2. Do not strain. Use the honey with the leaves incorporated. Enjoy by the spoonful; add to apple cider vinegar, marinades, or salad dressing; or make a tisane. If the sage leaves remain covered by the honey, the honey will keep for 1 year. It is not usually necessary to refrigerate it, but if the honey seems thin and liquid, refrigeration may be a good idea.

TO MAKE THE TISANE

1. Put the sage honey in a teapot, then cover with the boiling water. Cover with a lid, and steep for 20 minutes.

2. Pour the tisane through a tea strainer into a mug and enjoy.

NOTE: Make this honey with fresh sage leaves harvested from your patio pot, garden, or grocery produce section. The leaves are best picked on a hot, dry sunny day to gain the most aromatic oils from them.

Women's Decoction for Liver Health

MAKES: 4 cups

The liver plays a large role in hormonal health. Women's hormones are constantly changing, and if the liver is not working optimally, an excess of unnecessary hormones remains in the body and causes symptoms such as PMS, bloating, painful breasts, headaches, hair loss, insomnia, fatigue, and more. Schisandra and burdock support the liver. Schisandra is an adaptogen that normalizes liver functions. Burdock root is a bitter herb that increases the liver's metabolism and bile production. Licorice root protects the liver against damage from inflammation and oxidative stress. Ginger helps reduce inflammation and also increases blood circulation to carry these herbs throughout the body.

2 tablespoons dried schisandra berries

2 tablespoons dried burdock root

1 teaspoon dried ginger root (optional)

½ teaspoon dried licorice root (optional)

5 cups water

1. In a saucepot, combine the schisandra, burdock, and ginger and licorice, if desired. Cover with the water. Bring to a boil.

2. Reduce the heat to a simmer. Cover the pot and simmer for 30 minutes, or until the liquid has reduced to 4 cups. Remove from the heat. Steep for 20 minutes.

3. Pour the decoction through a tea strainer into a clean 32-ounce mason jar. Enjoy drinking throughout the day directly from the jar or poured into a mug. Store any remaining decoction in a covered jar in the refrigerator for up to 4 days.

NOTE: The ginger and licorice are added to this recipe for liver support and flavor, although you can omit them, if you prefer. The ginger will add spice and the licorice will add sweetness.

Summer Blossom Nervine Tisane

MAKES: 4 cups

This bright and floral tea will help smooth out your day no matter what stage of life you are in. The rose petals and linden blossoms are nervine in nature, meaning that they help nourish the nervous system, promote feelings of wellness, reduce stress, and ease irritability. These flowers are harvested in the same season; in many regions of North America, they bloom in the beginning of July, although you can also make this tisane with dried flowers.

½ cup fresh rose petals or ¼ cup dried

½ cup fresh linden blossoms or ¼ cup dried

4 cups boiling water
Honey, for serving (optional)

1. In a saucepot, combine the rose petals and linden blossoms. Cover with the boiling water. Cover and steep for 20 minutes.

2. Pour the tisane through a tea strainer into a clean 32-ounce mason jar.

3. Sweeten with a dash of honey, if desired. Drink the tisane straight from the jar, or pour into a mug to drink. Store any remaining tisane in a covered jar in the refrigerator for up to 2 days.

NOTE: I love to harvest the petals of wild *Rosa rugosa*, although any scented rose will work. Avoid roses from florists because the plants are treated with pesticides.

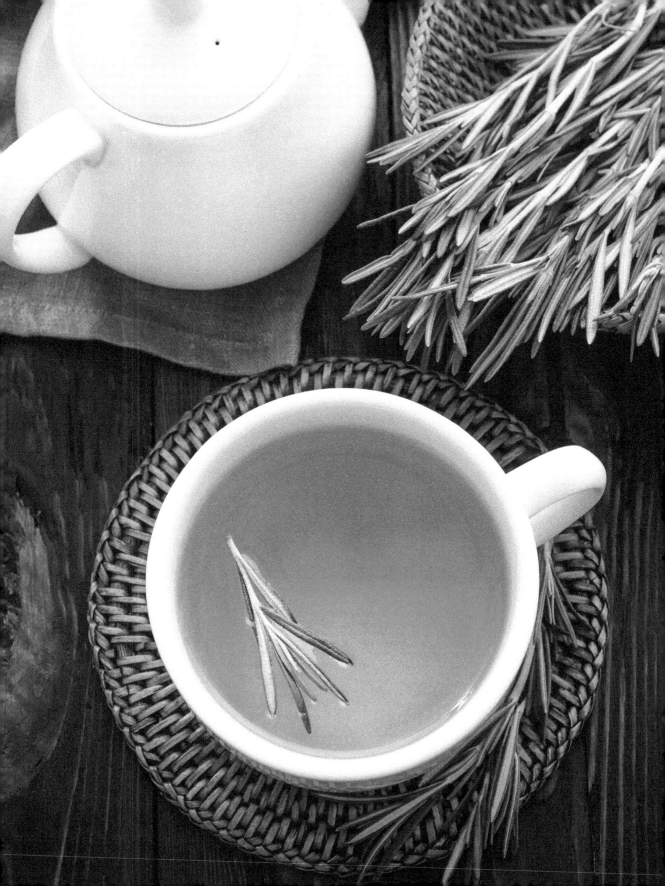

For the Nervous System and Brain Function

Let's explore how herbs support the health of the nervous system and brain function. In simple terms, the nervous system is a complex network that carries messages from the brain and spinal cord to various parts of the body. In this chapter, you will find infusions that can help relieve nerve pain and promote nerve repair, as well as beverages to help your brain fire on all cylinders.

You will also encounter recipes to nurture what is known as the gut-brain connection. Research is increasingly showing that healthy bacteria in the gut create hundreds of neuro-chemicals that the brain uses for physiological and mental processes, including learning, memory, and mood. In chapter 9, we'll focus on how herbs can support your emotional state, although many of the infusions in this chapter can help with that, too.

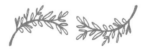

St. John's Wort Tincture to Ease Nerve Pain

MAKES: 2 cups

Although many people are familiar with St. John's wort (also known as St. Joan's wort) for its antidepressant effects, the herb also helps relieve nerve pain and heal damaged or pinched nerves. It can ease muscles that are stiff and sore from overexertion. To make this tincture, you need to use fresh flowers of the plant, whose botanical name is *Hypericum perforatum.* Remedies made from dried plant material will not work and will have the undesirable side effects of oversensitivity to the sun and increased risk of sunburn. The tincture has a unique floral flavor and a beautiful deep red color that is only extracted when fresh flowers are used.

2 cups fresh St. John's wort flowering tops

2 cups 100-proof vodka

1. Harvest the St. John's wort flowers and flower buds on a sunny day, at least 2 days after the last rain. The flowers bloom around summer solstice and through July.

2. Gently but tightly pack the flowers into a clean 16-ounce mason jar. There needs to be little air space between the flowers.

3. Fill the jar with the vodka. Cover with a tight lid, label, and let infuse for 6 weeks away from direct sunlight. The tincture will turn a beautiful deep red color on the first day of steeping.

4. Pour the tincture through a tea strainer into a clean measuring cup with a spout. Using a spoon, press the flowers to extract any remaining tincture.

5. Pour the tincture through a small funnel into 2 clean (8-ounce) Boston round amber bottles. Cover with tight lids and label. Tinctures keep indefinitely due to their alcohol content.

NOTE: St. John's/Joan's wort increases the speed at which the liver clears pharmaceutical drugs, especially when dried hypericum is used in supplement form. Because of this, speak with your pharmacist or doctor before working with Saint John's/Joan's wort in large therapeutic doses.

St. John's Nerve Repair Apple Spritzer

MAKES: 2 cups

This fun and simple apple spritzer uses St. John's wort tincture to make a flavorful beverage. It eases muscles that are sore from exercise or strain and repairs damaged nerves. This tincture can be purchased or made, as long as you have access to fresh St. John's/Joan's wort flowers. While St. John's wort is named as such due to its blooming around the Feast of St. John the Baptist in June, many prefer to call it St. Joan's wort in honor of Joan of Arc and the suffering she experienced at the stake. This is, in part, thanks to its ability to treat burns when infused in oil and applied topically.

1 teaspoon St. John's Wort Tincture to Ease Nerve Pain (page 109) or store-bought tincture

1 cup apple juice
1 cup bubbly water
1 teaspoon cinnamon powder
Ice, for serving

1 apple slice (optional)

1. In a pint glass, combine the tincture, apple juice, bubbly water, and cinnamon. Stir and add ice.

2. Garnish with an apple slice, if desired.

NOTE: St. John's/Joan's wort increases the speed at which the liver clears pharmaceutical drugs, especially when dried hypericum is used in supplement form. Because of this, speak with your pharmacist or doctor before working with St. John's/Joan's wort in large therapeutic doses. Begin with 1 teaspoon in this recipe, and increase as needed and advised to obtain your desired result.

Rest-and-Digest Infusion with Oat Straw and Chamomile

MAKES: 4 cups

This calming infusion helps activate the parasympathetic nervous system, which puts the body in rest-and-digest mode. Oat straw and astragalus root are both nervous-system tonics, improving its overall functioning. Oat straw provides important relaxing minerals such as calcium and magnesium. Chamomile both soothes the nerves and eases upset digestion. This beverage is made by combining a decoction of the astragalus and oat straw and a tisane of delicate chamomile flowers.

¼ cup dried oat straw
¼ cup dried astragalus
  root
5 cups water

4 teaspoons dried
  chamomile flowers or
  ¼ cup fresh

Honey, for serving
  (optional)

1. In a saucepot, combine the oat straw, astragalus, and water. Bring to a boil.

2. Reduce the heat to a simmer. Simmer for about 40 minutes, or until the liquid has reduced to about 4 cups. Remove from the heat.

3. Add the chamomile flowers. Cover the pot with a lid, and steep for 20 minutes.

4. Pour the infusion through a tea strainer into a clean 32-ounce mason jar.

5. Stir in honey, if desired. Enjoy the infusion straight from the jar, or pour into a mug to drink. Store any remaining infusion in a covered jar in the refrigerator for up to 2 days.

NOTE: This infusion is a great addition to smoothies.

Burdock Root Vinegar for the Brain-Gut Connection

MAKES: 2 cups

Increasingly, we are coming to understand that when our gut is healthy, our brain is, too. Burdock root–infused vinegar contains inulin, a starch that feeds the healthy bacteria in the gut. These microbes produce neurochemicals, such as serotonin and dopamine, that the brain needs to regulate thinking and mood. This recipe uses fresh burdock root. If you are not able to harvest your own, you can usually find it in a health-food store or Asian food store. Another name for burdock root is gobo root.

2 cups apple cider
   vinegar

2 cups diced scrubbed
   fresh burdock root

1. To pasteurize the vinegar, pour it into a nonmetal (Pyrex or ceramic-lined) pot and bring to a boil. Remove from the heat. Let cool to room temperature.

2. Put the burdock in a 16-ounce mason jar, then fill the jar to the top with the vinegar. Make sure all of the root is covered. Cover with a tight lid. If using a metal lid, lay a square of unbleached wax paper between the lid and the vinegar. For long-term storage of vinegar, use a plastic food-safe lid. Label the jar, and let infuse for 6 weeks away from direct sunlight. (The white sediment that forms is inulin.)

3. Pour the vinegar and inulin through a tea strainer into a measuring cup with a spout.

4. Remove the root from the jar. (The root can be used as a garnish for salads and other dishes.) Pour the vinegar and any remaining inulin back into the jar. This vinegar can be taken by the spoonful, added to drinks, or used as a base for a salad dressing. Pasteurized vinegars keep for 2 years or longer at room temperature.

NOTE: Before using the vinegar, shake the jar to mix in the inulin. This vinegar makes for a delicious salad dressing when combined with oil and honey. Mixing it in a blender makes a creamy dressing, due to the inulin.

Feed-the-Flora Burdock-Ginger Switchel

MAKES: 4 cups

A switchel is a refreshing drink made of water, a sweetener, lemon, apple cider vinegar, and ginger. It is believed to have been introduced from the West Indies to mainland America in the 17th century, becoming popular as an afternoon refreshment among farmers. This fun and tasty recipe promotes healthy gut flora, which, in turn, produce neurochemicals that support optimal brain function.

½ cup Burdock Root Vinegar for the Brain-Gut Connection (page 112)

2 tablespoons maple syrup or molasses

1 tablespoon freshly squeezed lemon juice

1 tablespoon Ginger Syrup to Ease an Upset Stomach (page 62) or store-bought ginger syrup

3 cups bubbly water

Ice, for serving

1. In a 32-ounce jar or pitcher, combine the vinegar, maple syrup, lemon juice, ginger syrup, and bubbly water. Stir or whisk to incorporate.

2. Pour the switchel into a glass over ice to drink. Store any remaining switchel in a covered jar in the refrigerator and drink over a day or two, after which it will lose its bubbly nature.

NOTE: You can make a larger switchel base of the burdock vinegar, sweetener, lemon juice, and ginger syrup, and store it in a Boston round amber bottle or another container in the refrigerator. It will store for several weeks if you do not add water to it. Combine with bubbly water and ice whenever you get a hankering.

Hawthorn Berry Nerve Decoction

MAKES: 4 cups

Hawthorn berries have been consumed as food and medicine for thousands of years. The berries are rich in bioflavonoids, which are anti-inflammatories important for nerve health. Chronic inflammation increases nerve pain and, in the long term, can cause nerve damage. Rounding out this recipe are nerve-nourishing oat tops, as well as cinnamon, which brings a hint of sweetness and helps circulate the remedy throughout your body.

5 tablespoons whole hawthorn berries
5 tablespoons whole dried oat tops

1 tablespoon cinnamon chips or 1 cinnamon stick
5 cups water

Honey, for serving (optional)

1. In a saucepot, combine the hawthorn, oat tops, cinnamon, and water. Bring to a boil.

2. Reduce the heat to a simmer. Simmer for 20 to 40 minutes, or until the liquid has reduced to about 4 cups. Remove from the heat. Cover the pot with a lid, and steep for 20 minutes.

3. Pour the decoction through a tea strainer into a clean 32-ounce mason jar.

4. Sweeten with honey, if desired. Enjoy straight from the jar, or pour into a mug to drink. Store any remaining decoction in a covered jar in the refrigerator for up to 2 days.

NOTE: This decoction can be sipped throughout the day and enjoyed on a regular basis.

Rosemary Tincture for Memory

MAKES: 2 cups

In Shakespeare's play *Hamlet*, Ophelia says, "There's rosemary, that's for remembrance." Recent research has shown this to be true, finding rosemary to be rich in antioxidants, which protect against free-radical damage in the brain that contributes to memory loss. Rosemary also increases blood flow to brain tissue, improving short-term recall, too. This tincture can be added to tea or bubbly water or taken by the dropperful.

2 cups chopped fresh rosemary leaves

2 cups 100-proof vodka

1. Put the rosemary in a clean 16-ounce mason jar, then fill the jar with the vodka. Cover with a tight lid, label and let infuse for 6 weeks away from direct sunlight.

2. Pour the tincture through a tea strainer into a clean measuring cup with a spout.

3. Pour the tincture through a small funnel into 2 clean (8-ounce) Boston round amber bottles. Cover with tight lids and label.

4. Take the tincture by the dropperful on its own, or add 1 teaspoon to a cup of bubbly water or tea. Tinctures keep indefinitely due to their alcohol content.

NOTE: Rosemary is easy to find in plant nurseries and can be grown in a pot outside or inside. When inside, it likes a sunny, moist location. Allow the soil to dry between watering. If the air is very dry, it will appreciate a water spritz on its leaves. In warm climates, rosemary is a perennial shrub. In cold climates with freezing winters, rosemary is an annual but can be overwintered inside.

Gingko Tincture for Brain Function

MAKES: 2 cups

Gingko is a classic herb for improving blood flow to the brain and enhancing brain function. It also contains antioxidants, although research is ongoing to determine if those in gingko may slow memory decline.

2 cups fresh yellow gingko leaves, chopped, or 1 cup dried, cut, and sifted leaves

2 cups 100-proof vodka

1. Gently but firmly pack the gingko leaves into a clean 16-ounce mason jar, then fill the jar with the vodka. Cover with a tight lid, label and let infuse for 6 weeks away from direct sunlight.

2. Pour the tincture through a tea strainer into a clean measuring cup with a spout.

3. Pour the tincture through a small funnel into 2 clean (8-ounce) Boston round amber bottles. Cover with tight lids and label. Take daily by the dropperful or added to a cup of tisane or coffee. Tinctures keep indefinitely due to their alcohol content.

NOTE: It is traditional to prepare gingko remedies with the yellow leaves that fall from the tree. Gingko is unique in that it drops all its leaves at one time. Some people combine yellow and green leaves in their remedies. If you do not have access to a gingko tree, you can purchase the dried leaves or the premade tincture. It is a common herbal remedy available commercially.

Memory-Boosting Hot Chocolate with Comfrey

MAKES: 4 cups

Comfrey leaf contains proteins that are important for short-term memory retention. This hot chocolate is a fun way to drink comfrey with the added benefits of feel-good theobromine found in cacao. The circulation-enhancing cinnamon in the recipe brings a hint of spice and sweetness to the drink.

2 cups Comfrey Infusion for Cell Repair (page 86)

1¾ cups milk or milk substitute

¼ cup bittersweet cacao powder

¼ cup sugar

1 teaspoon cinnamon powder

1. In a saucepot, combine the comfrey infusion and milk. Warm to a point just below a simmer.

2. Whisk in the cacao powder, sugar, and cinnamon until fully incorporated. Remove from the heat.

3. Pour the hot chocolate into a mug to enjoy. Any remaining beverage can be poured into a thermos to keep warm and be sipped throughout the day.

NOTE: Adjust the flavor to your liking by adding more cacao to make it more bitter or more sugar to make it sweeter. You can also melt a couple tablespoons of chocolate chips into the beverage for added decadence.

Green Tea with Rosemary for Focus

MAKES: 4 cups

Green tea has long been prized not only for its antioxidant effects but also as a refreshing pick-me-up thanks to its caffeine content, which helps awaken the mind and aid focus. This recipe pairs green tea with rosemary, which yields a beautiful bright and earthy flavor while increasing blood flow to the brain and promoting extra alertness.

2 tablespoons dried rosemary or ¼ cup fresh

1 tablespoon dried green tea or 2 tea bags

4 cups boiling water

1. Put the rosemary and green tea in a teapot, then cover with the boiling water. Cover with a lid, and steep for 20 minutes.

2. Pour the tea through a tea strainer into a clean 32-ounce mason jar. Enjoy straight from the jar, or pour into a mug to drink. Store any remaining tea in a covered jar in the refrigerator for up to 2 days.

NOTE: Rosemary is easy to grow in a pot. Bring it inside in the winter if you live in a place that freezes.

Ginger Elixir for Circulation to the Brain

MAKES: 2 cups

Ginger increases blood flow to the brain, carrying necessary nutrients and oxygen and thereby improving mental acuity. Ginger is a bright, spicy herb that helps clear winter depression, bringing cozy warmth to the body and mind. The stimulating nature of ginger enlivens the mind and spirit while relaxing the muscles of the body.

2 cups diced fresh
  ginger root

1½ cups 100-proof
  vodka

½ cup honey

1. Put the ginger in a clean 16-ounce mason jar, then fill the jar with the vodka. Pour in the honey. Cover the jar with a tight lid, label and let infuse for 6 weeks away from direct sunlight.

2. Pour the elixir through a tea strainer into a clean measuring cup with a spout.

3. Pour the elixir through a small funnel into 2 clean (8-ounce) Boston round amber bottles. Cover with tight lids and label. Take by the dropperful on its own, or add by the spoonful to tisanes, a shot glass of water, bubbly water, or cocktails. Elixirs keep indefinitely due to their alcohol content.

NOTE: Dried ginger root is much spicier than fresh, so if you only have access to dried, use ¾ cup for this recipe and use the elixir in smaller amounts.

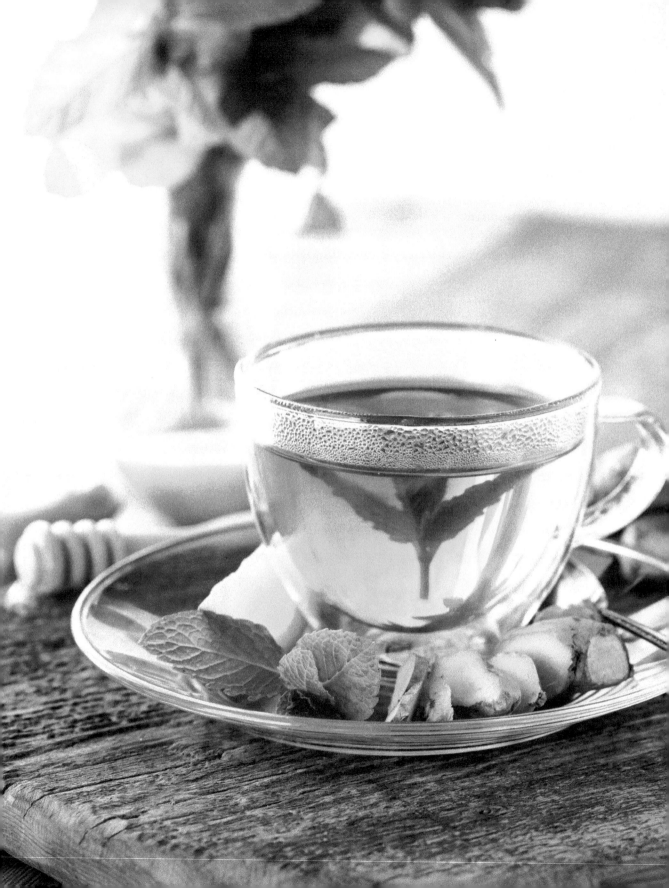

For Emotional Well-Being

In the busy modern world and with an array of competing responsibilities and challenges, it's no wonder that so many people find themselves on edge, fatigued, or low in spirits. Although herbal medicine won't fix underlying emotional problems, it can help us find calm in the midst of stress, boost our energy levels when weariness sets in, and lift our mood when it wanes.

Even the simple act of drinking one of these warming tisanes or refreshingly cool infusions will help foster better emotional well-being and mindfulness. Sipping these herbal beverages will let you take a moment out of the push and pull of your day so that you can reflect on life, connect with your senses, and appreciate the pleasures of the present moment.

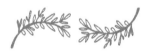

Calming Oat Straw Infusion

MAKES: 4 cups

Oat straw is a nutrient-rich herb that helps relieve anxiety and stress. It has an overall calming effect without being sedating. As a bonus, oat straw supports hormonal health and builds bone integrity. This infusion is sweet and slightly creamy. You can enjoy it cold poured over ice or heated with a dash of honey.

| 1 ounce dried, cut, and sifted oat straw | 4 cups boiling water | Honey, for serving (optional) |

1. Put the oat straw in a 32-ounce mason jar, then fill the jar to the top with the boiling water. Cover with a tight lid, and steep for a minimum of 4 hours or up to overnight.

2. Line the mouth of a ceramic drip coffee filter with a straining cloth. Pour the infusion through the filter into a clean 32-ounce mason jar.

3. Gather the corners of the straining cloth, and wring the cloth to squeeze as much liquid from the oat straw as you can.

4. Stir in honey to taste, if desired. Enjoy the infusion straight from the jar, or pour into a mug to drink. Store any remaining infusion in a covered jar in the refrigerator for up to 2 days.

NOTE: Drink up to 4 cups of oat straw infusion in one day, including it in a rotation of nourishing herbal infusions throughout the week. This infusion makes for a nice addition to a fruit-yogurt smoothie.

Milky Oat Top Tincture

MAKES: 2 cups

This tincture concentrates the pain-relieving and sedative properties of the oat plant from the milky seed heads. For this recipe, you will need to harvest fresh oat seed heads. Oat grass is an easy plant to grow and harvest, if you have space. It would even grow in a large pot, yielding enough milky tops for a small tincture.

3 cups fresh oat seed heads in their milky stage

2 cups 100-proof vodka

1. Harvest the oat seed heads in their "milky" stage between flowering and turning to seed. When you squeeze the top, a white milky substance should exude.

2. Put the oat seed heads and vodka in a blender. Blend until incorporated and bright green.

3. Pour the mixture into a clean 16-ounce mason jar (or larger, if needed). Cover with a tight lid, label, and infuse for 6 weeks away from direct sunlight.

4. Line the mouth of a ceramic drip coffee filter with a straining cloth. Pour the tincture through the filter into a clean 2-cup measuring cup with a spout.

5. Gather the corners of the straining cloth, and wring the cloth to squeeze as much liquid from the herbs as you can.

6. Pour the tincture through a small funnel into 2 clean (8-ounce) Boston round amber bottles. Cover with tight lids and label. Tinctures keep indefinitely due to their alcohol content.

NOTE: This tincture can be taken by the dropperful or added to an ounce of water and taken as needed. Start with small doses, and work your way up to a dose that gives you results. Given the sedating nature of the tincture, avoid driving and using machinery after consuming. If you cannot grow or forage your own milky oat tops, you can find a farm that has some available or you can purchase the tincture.

Soothing Double Oat Infusion

MAKES: 4 cups

This double oat infusion brings together the soothing properties of oat straw and milky oat tops—helping lower stress and acute anxiety, relieve pain, and ease you into rest and sleep. Milky oat top tincture can be purchased, or it can be made if you have access to fresh milky oat tops.

2 teaspoons Milky Oat Top Tincture (page 124) or store-bought tincture

4 cups Calming Oat Straw Infusion (page 123)

In a 32-ounce mason jar, combine the milky oat top tincture and oat straw infusion. Enjoy the infusion straight from the jar, or pour into a mug to drink. Store any remaining infusion in a covered jar in the refrigerator for up to 2 days.

NOTE: Given that the oat top tincture may be sedating, avoid driving and using machinery after taking until you know your tolerance level. You can add more flavor to the drink by adding a bit of apple juice or honey.

Flower Tisane for Frazzled Nerves

MAKES: 4 cups

Hawthorn and elderflowers are both great for soothing frazzled, frayed, or fried nerves. When life gets intense and overwhelming, allow these flowers to bring ease to your day. Hawthorn leaf and flower are also a tonic for the entire nervous system, improving its overall functioning and providing important minerals.

2 tablespoons dried, cut, and sifted hawthorn leaf and flower

2 tablespoons dried elderflowers

4 cups boiling water

Honey or Cooling Rose Petal Honey, for serving (page 88) (optional)

1. Put the hawthorn and elderflowers in a teapot, then cover with the boiling water. Cover with a lid, and steep for 20 minutes.

2. Pour the tisane through a tea strainer into a clean 32-ounce mason jar.

3. Sweeten with honey to taste, if desired. Enjoy the tisane straight from the jar, or pour into a mug to drink. Store any remaining tisane in a covered jar in the refrigerator for up to 2 days.

NOTE: These flowers bloom at different times of the summer, so you will not be able to make this tisane from fresh flowers. Hawthorn leaves and flowers are astringent. The sweet and slightly mucilaginous elderflowers are a nice complement and tone down the astringency of the hawthorn.

Lemon Balm Elixir to Ease Anxiety

MAKES: 2 cups

Lemon balm is a citrus-flavored mint that helps people who are jumpy, on edge, or experiencing prolonged stress. This elixir helps promote feelings of peace in times of chaos. This elixir can be added to bubbly water, cocktails with lemonade and vodka, or warm water with lemon. It can be taken by the spoonful or dropperful. For a stronger dose, enjoy it in a cordial glass with a splash of lemonade. For this recipe, harvest the top one-third of a lemon balm plant on a hot, sunny day.

2 cups fresh lemon balm leaves, finely chopped

1½ cups 100-proof vodka
½ cup honey

1. Put the lemon balm in a clean 16-ounce mason jar, then fill the jar with the vodka.

2. Pour in the honey. Make sure all of the herb is covered. Cover the jar with a tight lid, label, and let infuse for 6 weeks away from direct sunlight. The vodka and honey will meld over time. Shake the jar weekly or as often as you think of it.

3. Line the mouth of a ceramic drip coffee filter with a straining cloth. Pour the elixir through the filter into a clean measuring container with a spout.

4. Gather the corners of the straining cloth, and wring the cloth to squeeze as much liquid from the lemon balm as you can.

5. Pour the elixir through a small funnel into 4 clean (4-ounce) Boston round amber bottles. Cover with tight lids and label. Elixirs keep indefinitely due to their alcohol content.

NOTE: If you are prone to anxiety attacks, carry a small dropper bottle of this elixir with you and take a dropperful at the first sign of an attack. You should use fresh lemon balm leaves to make this elixir so that you can extract the volatile oils before the leaves dry. Lemon balm is easy to grow in a pot or garden. If you can't grow it, you can find a gardener friend or a farmer at a local farmers' market that has some.

Energizing Mint Fizz

MAKES: 4 cups

This bubbly mint beverage is a tasty antidote to tiredness and fatigue. The bright scent and taste of mint are refreshing for the senses, and studies have found that some of mint's natural compounds may have beneficial effects on energy levels and alertness. The addition of gingko and rosemary tinctures provide an extra boost for the brain. This can be sipped throughout the day, especially during times that require a lot of brain power and mental acuity. If you want a warm beverage, omit the bubbly water, add the tinctures to the mint tea when it is warm, and add a dash of honey, if desired.

1 tablespoon dried and crushed mint leaves
2 cups boiling water

1 teaspoon Gingko Tincture for Brain Function (page 116) or store-bought gingko tincture

1 teaspoon Rosemary Tincture for Memory (page 115) or store-bought rosemary tincture
2 cups bubbly water

1. Put the mint leaves in a teapot, then cover with the boiling water. Cover with a lid, and steep for 20 minutes.

2. Pour the tisane through a tea strainer into a clean 32-ounce mason jar. Let cool to room temperature.

3. Stir in the gingko tincture, rosemary tincture, and bubbly water. Enjoy the tisane straight from the jar, or pour into a glass over ice to drink. Store any remaining beverage in a covered jar in the refrigerator. It will only stay fizzy for 1 day, so if you want to store the beverage longer, wait to add the bubbly water to individual glasses instead of the entire tisane (which will last in a covered jar in the refrigerator for up to 3 days).

NOTE: There are a variety of mints that can be used, depending on what you have available or your preference. Peppermint is the most common. Chocolate mint, curly mint, apple mint, and spearmint are other varieties that you can experiment with. I think apple mint is delicious, and spearmint is a bit sweeter than peppermint, which is a bit spicier.

Triple Mint Tisane Pick-Me-Up

MAKES: 4 cups

This recipe brings together a trio of mint varieties in one refreshing tisane. It makes for a nice morning beverage or a midafternoon pick-me-up to keep you going. If you don't have these mint varieties on hand, you can replace them with any single variety of mint.

2 teaspoons dried apple mint or 2 tablespoons fresh

1 teaspoon dried chocolate mint or 2 tablespoons fresh

1 teaspoon dried curly mint or 2 tablespoons fresh

4 cups boiling water

1. Put the apple mint, chocolate mint, and curly mint in a teapot, then cover with the boiling water. Cover with a lid, and steep for 20 minutes.

2. Pour the tisane through a tea strainer into a clean 32-ounce jar. Enjoy straight from the jar, or pour into a mug to drink. Store any remaining tisane in a covered jar in the refrigerator for up to 3 days.

NOTE: There are a large variety of tasty mints that can easily be grown in a garden, on the edge of a lawn, or in pots. Most plant nurseries sell multiple varieties. You can add a tablespoon of fresh ginger to spice up this tisane, a dash of honey for sweetness, or a slice of lemon for a hint of sour.

Awakening Ginger-Mint Tisane

MAKES: 4 cups

Liven up your day with this spicy, refreshing, and classic combination of ginger and mint. These herbs will brighten the senses, get the blood flowing, and help keep your mind vibrant and tuned into your surroundings. Peppermint is a spicier mint than others (the clue is in the name). Peppermint combines with spicy ginger to add to the stimulating nature of this tisane.

4 teaspoons dried peppermint or ¼ cup fresh

2 teaspoons dried ginger root or ¼ cup fresh

4 cups boiling water

1. Put the peppermint and ginger in a teapot, then cover with the boiling water. Cover with a lid, and steep for 20 minutes.

2. Pour the tisane through a tea strainer into a clean 32-ounce mason jar. Enjoy straight from the jar, or pour into a mug to drink. Store any remaining tisane in a covered jar in the refrigerator for up to 3 days.

NOTE: Fresh ginger and dried peppermint are best for this tea, but work with what you have. You can add honey and lemon to the tisane, if desired.

Centering Tulsi Spritzer

MAKES: 4 cups

This is a fun and tasty bubbly drink that focuses on tulsi to help you feel more centered. Drink it on a regular basis to get the full benefit. This spritzer is especially beneficial during times of distress or low mood.

1 cup Tulsi and Mint Tisane for Emotional Balance (page 132), chilled

1 cup bubbly water
⅛ cup Tulsi Stress-Relief Syrup (page 133)

Ice, for serving
1 lemon wedge

1. In a large glass, combine the tisane, bubbly water, syrup, and a few ice cubes.

2. Squeeze a dash of lemon juice into the drink. Garnish with the lemon wedge. Store any remaining spritzer (with the lemon wedge removed, so that it does not become too sour) in a covered jar in the refrigerator for up to 24 hours.

NOTE: You can pour the drink into a thermos to keep it cool and sip throughout the day. If you're wanting to bring some herbal goodness to your next celebration, you can mix a glass of the spritzer with an ounce of vodka to make a cocktail.

Tulsi and Mint Tisane for Emotional Balance

MAKES: 4 cups

This warming tisane brings together the flavors and effects of tulsi and mint. The tulsi grounds and centers, while the mint refreshes and awakens. Any variety of mint can be used. Peppermint and spearmint are the two most common.

4 teaspoons dried tulsi   **4 teaspoons dried mint**   **4 cups boiling water**

1. Put the tulsi and mint in a teapot, then cover with the boiling water. Cover with a lid, and steep for 20 minutes.

2. Pour the tisane through a tea strainer into a clean 32-ounce mason jar. Enjoy straight from the jar, or pour into a mug to drink. Store any remaining tisane in a covered jar in the refrigerator for up to 3 days.

NOTE: This tisane can be poured into a glass over ice to enjoy cold for a delicious iced tea on a hot summer day. Both tulsi and mint are easy to grow in pots or a garden.

Tulsi Stress-Relief Syrup

MAKES: 2 cups

This tasty syrup supports health during stressful and adversarial times. It offers full body support, including immune-, digestive-, and nervous-system health. The syrup can be added to any beverage or smoothie. It can be enjoyed by the dropperful, spoonful, or shot glass.

1 tablespoon tulsi
1 cup boiling water

¾ cup honey or Cooling Rose Petal Honey (page 88)

1. Put the tulsi in a teapot, then cover with the boiling water. Cover with a lid, and steep for 45 minutes.

2. Pour the tisane through a tea strainer into a clean 16-ounce mason jar.

3. Add the honey, and stir to incorporate. Cover the jar, label, and store in the refrigerator for up to 4 months.

NOTE: You can enjoy this syrup by the spoonful throughout the day, especially during times of stress, or add it to tea, water, cocktails, bubbly water, or the Centering Tulsi Spritzer (page 131).

Relaxing Kava Infusion

MAKES: 4 cups

Kava is a plant found in the Pacific Islands and has been used for hundreds of years at ceremonies to foster camaraderie and feelings of well-being. It contains substances called kavapyrones that help you feel calm, relaxed, and happy. The infusion has a mild flavor and a slight numbing effect on the tongue.

1 ounce dried kava root   Honey, for serving
4 cups boiling water   (optional)

1. Put the kava root in a 32-ounce mason jar, then fill the jar to the top with the boiling water. Cover with a tight lid, and steep for a minimum of 4 hours or overnight.

2. Line the mouth of a ceramic drip coffee filter with a straining cloth. Pour the infusion through the filter into a clean 32-ounce mason jar.

3. Gather the corners of the straining cloth, and wring the cloth to squeeze as much liquid from the kava root as you can.

4. Stir in honey to taste, if desired. Enjoy the infusion directly from the jar, or pour into a mug to drink. Store any remaining infusion in a covered jar for up to 2 days in the refrigerator.

NOTE: In large enough amounts, kava may be sedating enough that you should avoid driving or operating heavy machinery while feeling its effects. It may interact with psychiatric and pain medications. Do not use kava leaf, as it can damage the liver.

Elixir for Better Sleep and Pain Relief

MAKES: 2 cups

This elixir is both a pain reliever and a sedative to aid sleep. The desired effect depends on how much you take and your sensitivity to the blend. Start with low doses of 5 to 10 drops of the elixir, and work your way up from there. Low doses are more for pain relief, whereas larger doses will have more of a sedative effect.

1 cup chopped fresh passionflower flower and leaf or ⅓ cup dried

1 cup chopped California poppy whole plant or ⅓ cup dried

1½ cups 100-proof vodka
½ cup honey

1. Put the passionflower and poppy in a clean 16-ounce mason jar, then fill the jar with the vodka.

2. Pour in the honey. Make sure the herbs are fully covered. Cover the jar with a tight lid, label and let infuse for 6 weeks away from direct sunlight.

3. Line the mouth of a ceramic drip coffee filter with a straining cloth. Pour the elixir through the filter into a clean 16-ounce mason jar.

4. Gather the corners of the straining cloth, and wring the cloth to squeeze as much liquid from the herbs as you can.

5. Take the elixir by the drop or dropperful as needed. Elixirs keep indefinitely due to their alcohol content.

NOTE: You can add the elixir in the same recommended amounts to a glass over bubbly water to make a refreshing beverage.

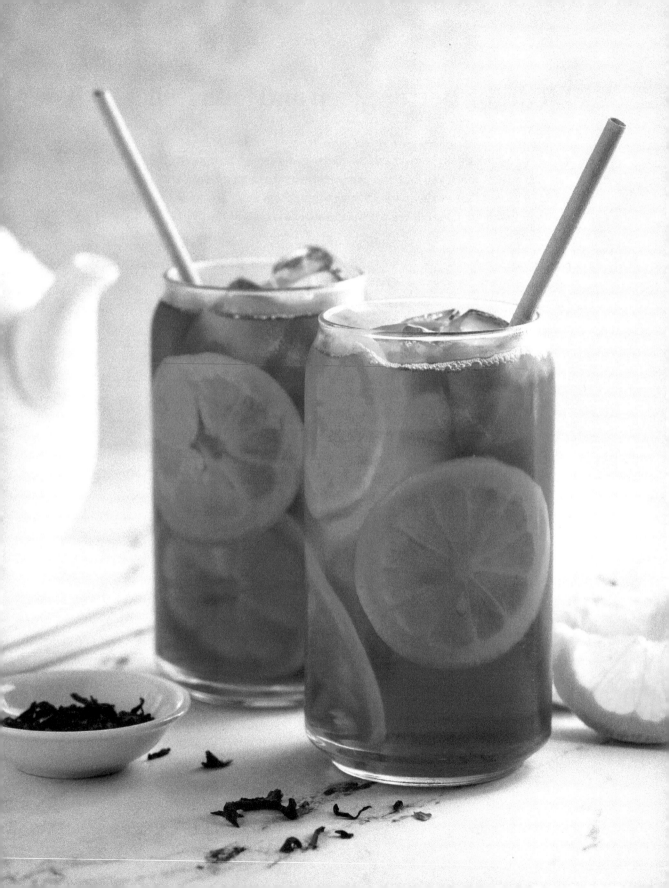

For the Cardiovascular System

Together, the heart and blood vessels make up the cardiovascular system, which circulates oxygen, blood, and nutrients around the body for optimal performance. Although lifestyle factors such as exercise and overall diet are central to heart health, there are numerous herbs that can bring a little boost to our cardiac health.

Studies have linked certain herbs to lowering blood pressure, delivering cardiac-protecting antioxidants, and easing stress that contributes to heart complications, among other benefits. The recipes in this chapter showcase some of the superstars of herbal heart health, including hibiscus, hawthorn, oat straw, rose, cinnamon, cacao, mint, astragalus, motherwort, tulsi, and chamomile.

If you take medication for a cardiovascular condition, be sure to consult with a medical professional about any possible interactions different herbs may have with your medication.

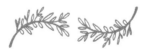

Hibiscus and Mint Tisane for Heart Health

MAKES: 4 cups

Hibiscus is prized in infusions not only for its ruby red color and tart flavor but also as a true tonic for the heart. Studies have linked it to lowering blood pressure, improving healthy cholesterol levels, and delivering antioxidants that help reduce the risk of heart disease. Hibiscus is complemented here by the bright flavor of mint.

4 teaspoons dried hibiscus flowers

4 teaspoons dried and crushed mint leaves

4 cups boiling water

1. Put the hibiscus flowers and mint leaves in a teapot, then cover with the boiling water. Cover with a lid, and steep for 20 minutes.

2. Pour the tisane through a tea strainer into a clean 32-ounce mason jar. Enjoy straight from the jar, or pour into a mug to drink. Store any remaining tisane in a covered jar in the refrigerator for up to 4 days.

NOTE: Hibiscus flowers commonly sold in herbal stores are the calyxes of the species *Hibiscus sabdariffa*. These flowers are best for making infusions. They are hard, deep-red pieces that look like petals but are in fact the outside layer of the flower buds.

Hibiscus and Strawberry Shrub

MAKES: 2 cups

This recipe delivers the heart-healthy benefit of hibiscus in a sweet-tart herbal shrub (drinking vinegar) that can be enjoyed by the spoonful, by the shot glass, in a cocktail, in ice water, or in bubbly water.

1½ cups apple cider vinegar

¼ cup dried hibiscus flowers

½ cup chopped frozen strawberries

½ cup honey

1. To pasteurize the vinegar, pour it into a nonmetal (Pyrex or ceramic-lined) pot and bring to a boil. Remove from the heat. Let cool to room temperature.

2. Put the hibiscus and strawberries in a 16-ounce mason jar, then fill the jar with the vinegar.

3. Pour in the honey. Make sure the flowers and fruit are fully covered. Cover the jar with a tight lid. If using a metal lid, lay a square of unbleached wax paper between the lid and the vinegar. For long-term storage of vinegar, use a plastic food-safe lid. Label the jar, and let infuse for 6 weeks away from direct sunlight.

4. Line the mouth of a ceramic drip coffee filter with a straining cloth. Pour the shrub through the filter into a measuring cup with a spout.

5. Pour the shrub through a small funnel into 2 clean (8-ounce) Boston round amber bottles. Cover with plastic lids and label. Enjoy by the spoonful, in a cup of bubbly water, or in a warm mug of water. Made with pasteurized vinegar, shrubs will keep for up to 1 year at room temperature.

NOTE: Frozen berries extract better than fresh berries because their cell walls have been broken open in the freezing process. This allows more nutrients, antioxidants, and flavor to be released readily. Once the fruit is strained, it can be enjoyed on yogurt, ice cream, smoothies, or baked treats.

Four-Herb Heart Tonic

MAKES: 4 cups

Cardiovascular disease of varying types is a leading health concern in the modern world. For this reason alone, it is important to support the aging heart with herbal heart tonics. Heart tonics strengthen and improve the normal functioning of the heart and cardiovascular system as a whole. The herbs in this recipe offer necessary bioflavonoids, vitamins, and minerals that build heart health, strength, and flexibility. To gain their long-term benefits, consume these herbs on a regular basis.

¼ cup dried hawthorn berries

¼ cup dried oat straw

¼ cup dried rose hips

¼ cup dried astragalus root

5 cups water

Honey, for serving (optional)

1. In a saucepot, combine the hawthorn, oat straw, rose hips, astragalus root, and water. Bring to a boil.

2. Reduce the heat to a simmer. Cover the pot and simmer for 30 minutes, or until the liquid has reduced to about 4 cups. Remove from the heat. Steep for 20 minutes.

3. Pour the tonic through a tea strainer into a clean 32-ounce mason jar.

4. Stir in honey to taste, if desired. Enjoy the tonic straight from the jar, or pour into a mug to drink. Store any remaining tonic in a covered jar in the refrigerator for up to 2 days.

NOTE: This decoction is a hydrating cold beverage when poured over ice.

Hot Chocolate with Cinnamon for Better Blood Flow

MAKES: 2 cups

Although chocolate is not often thought to be synonymous with good health, realistically, its principal ingredient, cacao, offers an impressively long list of benefits for the cardiovascular system. The secret? It is rich in flavonoids that help reduce blood pressure, lower cholesterol, and improve the functioning of blood vessels. This recipe includes cinnamon, which also helps improve blood flow through the body.

1¾ cups milk or your preferred milk substitute

1 tablespoon cinnamon powder

¼ cup bittersweet cacao powder

2 tablespoons sugar

1. In a saucepot, combine the milk and cinnamon. Heat to just below simmering.

2. Whisk in the cacao powder and sugar until fully incorporated. Remove from the heat.

3. Pour the hot chocolate into a mug to drink.

NOTE: The sugar and cinnamon amounts can be adjusted to your taste preference.

Antioxidant-Rich Syrup with Hawthorn and Rose

MAKES: 2 cups

Hawthorn berries and rose hips are two wild fruits that support heart functions with antioxidants as well as nutrition from an array of necessary vitamins and minerals. This syrup concentrates their medicinal benefit into a tasty daily heart tonic.

2 cups water

¼ cup fresh hawthorn berries or 2 tablespoons dried

¼ cup fresh rose hips or 2 tablespoons dried

1 cup honey or Cooling Rose Petal Honey (page 88)

1. In a saucepot, combine the water, hawthorn berries, and rose hips. Bring to a boil.

2. Reduce the heat to a simmer. Simmer for about 1 hour, or until the liquid has reduced by half. Remove from the heat.

3. Line the mouth of a ceramic drip coffee filter with a straining cloth. Pour the decoction through the filter into a clean 16-ounce mason jar.

4. Add the honey, and stir until fully incorporated.

5. Pour the syrup through a small funnel into 2 clean (8-ounce) Boston round amber bottles. Cover with tight lids and label. The syrup will keep for up to 6 months in the refrigerator.

NOTE: This syrup can be enjoyed by the spoonful or shot glass–full or can be added to bubbly water, tisane, juice, or cocktails. A tablespoon of hibiscus flowers can be added to the herbs for the decoction, for color, flavor, and added health benefit.

Herbal Cordial for Cardiac Protection

MAKES: 2 cups

A cordial is a sweet herbal liqueur in which alcohol is used to concentrate a plant's medicine. Cordials are traditionally designed for heart health. In fact, "cordial" is a synonym for "heartfelt" and derives from the Latin word "cor," which means "heart." This recipe showcases cacao, rose, and motherwort, a trio of heart-healthy herbs rich in antioxidants known to help protect cardiac health. Motherwort is known to increase the capillary bed around the heart, allowing for more blood to easily be pumped through the heart.

¼ cup cacao nibs

1 cup fresh chopped rose petals or ½ cup dried

½ cup fresh chopped motherwort leaves and flowering tops or ¼ cup dried

1½ cups 100-proof vodka

½ cup honey

1. Put the cacao nibs, rose petals, and motherwort in a clean 16-ounce mason jar, then fill the jar with the vodka.

2. Pour in the honey. Make sure that all the herbs are covered. Cover the jar with a tight lid, label and let infuse for 6 weeks away from direct sunlight.

3. Line the mouth of a ceramic drip coffee filter with a straining cloth. Pour the cordial through the filter into a clean 2-cup measuring cup with a spout.

4. Pour the cordial through a small funnel into 2 clean (8-ounce) Boston round amber bottles. Cover with tight lids and label. Enjoy by the spoonful or shot glass–full or added to bubbly water or cocktails. Cordials will keep for many years due to their alcohol content.

NOTE: This cordial tastes best with fresh rose petals and fresh motherwort. Although you can use dried rose petals, if needed, dried motherwort will bring a bitter flavor.

Hawthorn and Cinnamon Tisane to Regulate Blood Pressure

MAKES: 4 cups

Both cinnamon bark and hawthorn leaves and flowers normalize blood-pressure levels when consumed on a regular basis. Cinnamon dilates blood vessels and reduces unhealthy cholesterol to improve blood flow. Hawthorn is a tonic to the cardiovascular system and the heart itself. As a tonic, it improves the overall functioning of the system. It can take a few months to a couple years of drinking hawthorn tisane before you notice substantial changes in the health of your blood-pressure levels.

2 teaspoons cinnamon powder

¼ cup dried hawthorn leaves and flowers

4 cups boiling water

1. Put the cinnamon and hawthorn in a teapot, then cover with the boiling water. Cover with a lid, and steep for 20 minutes.

2. Pour the tisane through a tea strainer into a clean 32-ounce mason jar. Enjoy straight from the jar, or pour into a mug to drink. Store any remaining tisane in a covered jar in the refrigerator for up to 2 days.

NOTE: You can use a cinnamon stick or chips instead of powder. Add it to the water as it boils to release its flavor before pouring them both into the teapot.

Heart-Friendly Wine Infusion with Hawthorn and Rose

MAKES: 4 cups

For folks who already enjoy a glass of wine in the evening, why not add heart-healthy herbs to your glass? Not only does wine make for a great menstruum (solvent) for infusing herbs, but also it contains anthocyanins that are beneficial for heart health. In this remedy, we add supporting herbs and berries for additional flavor and cardiac benefit.

1 (25-ounce) bottle pinot noir or another light red wine you prefer

1 cup chopped fresh hawthorn berries or ½ cup dried, coarsely ground

1 cup chopped fresh rose petals or ½ cup dried

1 cup chopped frozen strawberries

1 cinnamon stick (optional)

1. Put the wine, hawthorn berries, rose petals, strawberries, and cinnamon, if desired, in a 32-ounce mason jar. Lay a square of unbleached parchment paper between the lid and the liquid. Cover with a tight lid, label, and let infuse for at least 3 days away from direct sunlight.

2. Line the mouth of a ceramic drip coffee filter with a straining cloth. Pour the infusion through the filter into a clean 32-ounce mason jar.

3. Gather the corners of the straining cloth, and wring the cloth to squeeze as much liquid from the herbs and fruit as you can.

4. Pour the infusion through a funnel into a clean empty wine bottle. Cap with a cork, and label. Enjoy 1 glass per evening. The infusion will keep for 1 week.

NOTE: For a richer flavor, infuse the herbs into the wine for 7 days, which will also impart stronger medicinal benefit. When it's ready to serve, you can turn it into a wine spritzer by adding some ice, bubbly water, and a fresh strawberry.

Hawthorn Berry Cordial with Cinnamon and Ginger

MAKES: 2 cups

This cordial brings together hawthorn berry, cinnamon, and ginger for a spicy, fruity tonic for the heart. It is especially beneficial for people who want to improve circulation to the extremities and lower blood pressure.

1½ cups fresh chopped hawthorn berries or ¾ cup dried, coarsely ground

¼ cup fresh chopped ginger root
1 tablespoon cinnamon chips or 1 cinnamon stick

1½ cups 100-proof vodka
½ cup honey

1. Put the hawthorn berries, ginger, and cinnamon chips in a clean 16-ounce mason jar, then fill the jar with the vodka.

2. Pour in the honey. Make sure all the herbs are covered. Cover the jar with a tight lid, label and let infuse for at least 6 weeks away from direct sunlight.

3. Line the mouth of a ceramic drip coffee filter with a straining cloth. Pour the cordial through the filter into a clean 2-cup measuring cup with a spout.

4. Pour the cordial through a small funnel into 2 clean (8-ounce) Boston round amber bottles. Cover with tight lids and label. Enjoy by the spoonful or shot glass–full or added to bubbly water or cocktails. Cordials keep for several years due to their alcohol content.

NOTE: If you want to make this cordial spicy, use 2 tablespoons of dried ginger instead of ¼ cup of fresh ginger.

Tulsi and Chamomile Tisane to Ease the Heart

MAKES: 4 cups

It's no secret that chronic stress is a key risk factor for heart complications. There are many important considerations in pursuing a less stressful lifestyle, and this warming tisane makes for a soothing addition to your routine. It combines the benefits of tulsi and chamomile, both known to calm the nervous system. It is especially pleasant in the evening to help prepare for a restful sleep.

2 teaspoons dried tulsi leaves and flowering tops or 2 tablespoons fresh

2 teaspoons dried chamomile flowers or 2 tablespoons fresh

4 cups boiling water

1. Put the tulsi and chamomile in a teapot, then cover with the boiling water. Cover with a lid, and steep for 20 minutes.

2. Pour the tisane through a tea strainer into a clean 32-ounce mason jar. Enjoy straight from the jar, or pour into a mug to drink. Store any remaining tisane in a covered jar in the refrigerator for up to 3 days.

NOTE: You can pour this tisane into a thermos to keep warm and enjoy throughout a stressful day. Either one of the herbs is a nice tea on its own. Simply double the amount of the herb in the recipe. Sweeten with a dash of honey and a slice of lemon, if desired.

Rooibos and Rose Heart Tonic

MAKES: 4 cups

This tonic is a combination of rose hip decoction and rose petal and rooibos tisane to improve overall heart function. It can be consumed weekly to tone the heart and normalize blood pressure over time. Rooibos is a plant native to South Africa and is often called "African red tea" or "red bush tea." It has a pleasant nutty-vanilla taste and imparts a beautiful red color to water it infuses into. Rooibos is loaded with antioxidants that support the heart and help normalize blood pressure and cholesterol. Rose is a gentle heart tonic that offers a full range of vitamins, minerals, and antioxidants.

¼ cup dried rose hips

5 cups water

4 teaspoons dried rose petals

4 teaspoons dried rooibos

Honey, for serving (optional)

1. In a saucepot, combine the rose hips and water. Bring to a boil.

2. Reduce the heat to a simmer. Simmer for about 30 minutes, or until the liquid has reduced to about 4 cups. Remove from the heat.

3. Add the rose petals and rooibos. Cover the pot with a lid, and steep for 20 minutes.

4. Pour the tonic through a tea strainer into a clean 32-ounce mason jar.

5. Stir in honey to taste, if desired. Enjoy the tonic from the jar, or pour into a mug to drink. Store any remaining tonic in a covered jar in the refrigerator for up to 4 days.

NOTE: Rooibos is tasty and can be enjoyed in a tea by itself. Simply steep 1 teaspoon per cup of boiling water for 20 minutes. Rooibos is easy to find in tea bags at your local health-food store or online.

Happy Heart Rooibos Chai

MAKES: 4 cups

The heart-tonic and blood pressure–modulating benefits of rooibos combine with warming circulatory-enhancing herbs to make a delicious beverage. The chai spices are decocted and then once they are removed from the heat, the rooibos is added to steep. Add your preference of milk and a bit of honey to sweeten, and this beverage will be a mainstay in your herbal beverage repertoire.

2 cinnamon sticks
4 teaspoons clove buds
6 fresh ginger slices

8 cardamom pods, crushed
5 cups water
2 tablespoons rooibos

Honey, for serving (optional)
Milk or half-and-half, for serving (optional)

1. In a saucepot, combine the cinnamon, clove buds, ginger, cardamom, and water. Bring to a boil.

2. Reduce the heat to a simmer. Simmer for about 30 minutes, or until the liquid has reduced to about 4 cups. Remove from the heat.

3. Add the rooibos, cover the pot with a lid, and steep for 20 minutes.

4. Pour the chai through a tea strainer into a clean 32-ounce mason jar.

5. Add honey and milk to taste, if desired. Enjoy the chai straight from the jar, or pour into a mug to drink.

NOTE: The chai spices are a popular combination that you can easily purchase pre-mixed and in tea bags at your local health-food store or online, if you would rather not blend your own.

Schisandra Berry Heart Syrup

MAKES: 2 cups

In China, the schisandra berry is known as the "five-flavor fruit" because it possesses all five of the basic flavors of Chinese herbal medicine: sweet, sour, bitter, salty, and spicy. Rich in bioflavonoids, it is known to help improve circulation and overall heart health, and has also been linked to improved liver function. This recipe makes a full-flavored syrup that tastes best diluted in small amounts into bubbly water, cocktails, hot water, dressings, and marinades.

1 cup dried schisandra berries

2 cups water
1 cup honey

1. Put the berries in a saucepot, then cover with the water. Bring to a boil.

2. Reduce the heat to a simmer. Simmer for about 40 minutes, or until the liquid has reduced by half. Remove from the heat.

3. Line the mouth of a ceramic drip coffee filter with a straining cloth. Pour the decoction through the filter into a clean 16-ounce mason jar.

4. Add the honey, and stir until fully incorporated.

5. Pour the syrup through a small funnel into 2 clean (8-ounce) Boston round amber bottles. Cover with tight lids and label. The syrup will keep in the refrigerator for up to 4 months.

NOTE: Schisandra has been used in traditional Chinese medicine for thousands of years and is considered beneficial to qi, the life force or energy inherent in all living things.

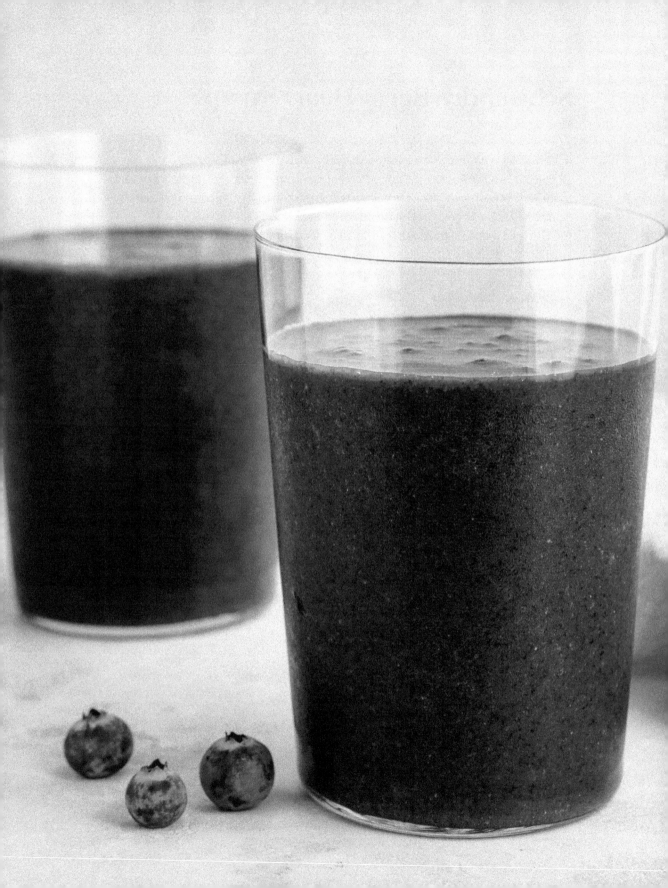

For Maintaining a Resilient Body

Diet, exercise, and other lifestyle factors are certainly key when it comes to our overall health, but herbal medicine is a powerful ally to maintain lifelong vitality and protect against chronic conditions. The herbs throughout this chapter—including astragalus, schisandra, eleuthero, ginger, and green tea, among others—have been chosen for a variety of qualities. There are adaptogens that counteract the effects of stress in the body; antioxidants believed to clear the body of cell-damaging free radicals; and anti-inflammatories known to reduce chronic inflammation, which is increasingly linked to a range of serious diseases. Along with these are nutritive herbs that provide all-around nourishment to help sustain long-term wellness.

If I could suggest just one herbal routine to maintain health, it would be the Rotation of Herbal Infusions for Resiliency (page 155). It is a simple and enjoyable self-care practice that can yield incredible long-term benefits.

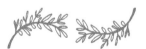

Rotation of Herbal Infusions for Resiliency

MAKES: 4 cups

This is not really a single recipe but rather a rotation of five different herbal infusions. Although you can find individual infusions in this book that showcase the five herbs in this recipe—stinging nettle leaf, comfrey leaf, oat straw, linden, and red clover blossoms—I have provided this rotation because I truly believe it may be the most valuable self-care practice you can take up as a newcomer to herbalism. Simply choose one herb to infuse one day, then another herb the following day, until you have worked through all five herbs—then start again.

1 ounce chosen dried herb (stinging nettle leaf, comfrey leaf, oat straw, linden, or red clover blossoms)

4 cups boiling water

1. Each day, choose one herb to brew.

2. Put your chosen herb in a 32-ounce mason jar, then fill the jar to the top with the boiling water. Cover with a tight lid, and steep for a minimum of 4 hours or up to overnight.

3. Line the mouth of a ceramic drip coffee filter with a straining cloth. Pour the infusion through the filter into a clean 32-ounce mason jar. Enjoy straight from the jar, or put in a thermos to carry with you to finish throughout the day.

NOTE: I especially recommend this rotation for pregnant or nursing women to boost the health of both mother and child.

Stamina-Building Infusion with Eleuthero

MAKES: 4 cups

Eleuthero, otherwise known as Siberian ginseng, is a mild-tasting herb native to Russia, Japan, Korea, and China. Though it is not related to ginseng, it has similar properties and therefore bears its name. It is an adaptogen herb that has been found to provide energy, build stamina, and promote resilience.

1 ounce dried eleuthero root   4 cups boiling water

1. Put the eleuthero in a 32-ounce mason jar, then fill the jar to the top with the boiling water. Cover with a tight lid, and steep for a minimum of 4 hours or up to overnight.

2. Line the mouth of a ceramic drip coffee filter with a straining cloth. Pour the infusion through the filter into a clean 32-ounce mason jar.

3. Gather the corners of the straining cloth, and wring the cloth to squeeze as much liquid from the eleuthero as you can.

4. Enjoy the infusion straight from the jar, or pour into a glass over ice to drink. Store any remaining infusion in a covered jar in the refrigerator for up to 2 days.

NOTE: Eleuthero has a mild flavor. If you want to jazz up this infusion, pour it into a mug, heat it up, and add your favorite herbal tea bag to it. Eleuthero can be added as a sixth herb to the Rotation of Herbal Infusions for Resiliency (page 155) for more variety.

Adapt and Flow Herbal Smoothie

MAKES: 4 cups

This smoothie is a great way to start the day, building energy, stamina, immunity, and resiliency thanks to a trio of herbs—schisandra berry, eleuthero, and astragalus—prized by herbalists for their apoptogenic qualities. You can enjoy the smoothie for breakfast or carry it with you in a thermos to drink throughout the day.

1 teaspoon schisandra berry powder

1 tablespoon eleuthero powder

1 tablespoon astragalus powder

1 tablespoon honey or Schisandra Berry Heart Syrup (page 151)

1 cup chopped frozen bananas

½ cup frozen blueberries

2 cups whole-milk plain yogurt, plus more as needed

1½ cups lemonade or Calming Oat Straw Infusion (page 123), plus more as needed

1. Put the schisandra berry powder, eleuthero powder, astragalus powder, honey, bananas, blueberries, yogurt, and lemonade in a blender. Blend until smooth.

2. Add more lemonade or oat straw infusion to make the smoothie thinner or more yogurt to make it thicker to yield your desired consistency.

3. Pour the smoothie into a glass and enjoy. Store any remaining smoothie in a covered jar in the refrigerator for up to 2 days.

NOTE: You can change the fruit and juice, depending on what you have on hand.

Spiced Medicinal Mushroom Tea

MAKES: 4 cups

The earthy umami of mushroom flavor blends well with spices found in chai, a popular tea in India. Not only do mushrooms benefit a range of body systems, but they are also the highest dietary source of ergothioneine, a unique and effective antioxidant and cellular protector that has been linked to lowering the risk of cancer.

6 cups water
6 chopped dried or fresh shiitake mushrooms

¼ cup chopped dried or fresh maitake mushrooms
1 teaspoon cinnamon chips or ½ cinnamon stick

1 teaspoon dried ginger
4 crushed cardamom pods
4 whole cloves
1 teaspoon fennel seeds

1. In a saucepot, combine the water, shiitake mushrooms, and maitake mushrooms. Bring to a boil.

2. Reduce the heat to low. Cover the pot, and simmer for 1 hour.

3. Remove the lid, and continue to simmer until the liquid has reduced to about 4 cups.

4. Add the cinnamon, ginger, cardamom, cloves, and fennel seeds. Partially cover the pot, and simmer for 20 minutes. Remove from the heat. Let cool.

5. Line the mouth of a ceramic drip coffee filter with a straining cloth. Pour the tea through the filter into a clean 32-ounce mason jar. Enjoy from the jar, or pour into a mug to drink.

NOTE: Other mushrooms you can substitute into the mix include fresh or dried turkey tail mushrooms or dried reishi mushrooms.

Antioxidant Oxymel with Rosemary and Thyme

MAKES: 2 cups

Rosemary and thyme are two herbs in the vast mint family of plants. They are loaded with nutritious minerals, vitamins, and antioxidant components, helping promote resilience throughout the body. This recipe brings them together in an oxymel, which is a combination of apple cider vinegar and honey. The vinegar is an effective menstruum (solvent) for extracting minerals and medicinal qualities from herbs.

1½ cups apple cider vinegar	1 cup fresh rosemary leaves	1 cup fresh thyme leaves
		½ cup honey

1. To pasteurize the vinegar, pour it into a nonmetal (Pyrex or ceramic-lined) pot and bring to a boil. Remove from the heat. Let cool to room temperature.

2. Put the rosemary and thyme in a 16-ounce mason jar, then fill the jar with the vinegar.

3. Pour in the honey. Make sure the herbs are totally covered. Cover the jar with a tight lid. If using a metal lid, lay a square of unbleached wax paper between the lid and the vinegar. For long-term storage of vinegar, use a plastic food-safe lid. Label the jar, and let infuse for 6 weeks away from direct sunlight.

4. Line the mouth of a ceramic drip coffee filter with a straining cloth. Pour the oxymel through the filter into a 2-cup measuring cup with a spout.

5. Pour the oxymel through a small funnel into 2 clean (8-ounce) Boston round amber bottles. Cover with tight plastic lids and label. When made with pasteurized vinegar, oxymels keep indefinitely.

NOTE: This sweet and savory oxymel can be taken by the spoonful, stirred into a cup of bubbly water over ice, or stirred into a mug of hot water. It is also a flavorful ingredient for marinades and salad dressings.

Antioxidant Wild-Berry Shrub

MAKES: 4 cups

A shrub is a combination of vinegar, honey (or sugar), and fruit. Vinegar extracts the nutrition and antioxidants from the fruit. The honey sweetens and balances the sour of the vinegar. Shrubs can be enjoyed by the spoonful or shot glass–full. They can be added to bubbly water, juice, tea, or cocktails.

3 cups apple cider vinegar

1 cup fresh chopped hawthorn berries or ½ cup dried

2 cups fresh chopped rose hips or 1 cup dried

1 cup elderberries or ½ cup dried

1 cup honey

1. To pasteurize the vinegar, pour it into a nonmetal (Pyrex or ceramic-lined) pot and bring to a boil. Remove from the heat. Let cool to room temperature.

2. Put the hawthorn berries, rose hips, and elderberries in a 32-ounce mason jar, then fill the jar with the vinegar.

3. Pour in the honey. Make sure the berries are totally covered. Cover the jar with a tight lid. If using a metal lid, lay a square of unbleached wax paper between the lid and the vinegar. For long-term storage of vinegar, use a plastic food-safe lid. Label the jar, and let infuse for 6 weeks away from direct sunlight.

4. Line the mouth of a ceramic drip coffee filter with a straining cloth. Pour the shrub through the filter into a 4-cup measuring cup with a spout.

5. Pour the shrub through a small funnel into 4 clean (8-ounce) Boston round amber bottles. Cover with tight plastic lids and label. Take by the spoonful or shot glass–full on its own or stirred into bubbly water over ice or hot water. When made with pasteurized vinegar, shrubs will keep indefinitely.

NOTE: This shrub can be made with just one of the berries instead of all three. Adjust the amount so the total amount of berries is the same. You may also replace them with different wild or cultivated berries. When using rose hips, make sure that the straining cloth has a tight weave so that none of the hip hairs get through the cloth and into the shrub. The hairs can irritate the throat and digestive tract.

Antioxidant-Rich Mediterranean Herb Tisane

MAKES: 4 cups

Oregano, thyme, rosemary, and sage are familiar favorites in Mediterranean cooking, but did you know that they are also rich in cell-protecting antioxidants? On top of that, they also possess antibacterial and antimicrobial qualities that help ward against infection. This recipe produces a savory tisane, but you can add honey for sweetness or a lemon for a slightly tart flavor.

1 teaspoon dried oregano or 1 tablespoon chopped fresh leaves

1 teaspoon dried thyme or 1 tablespoon chopped fresh leaves

1 teaspoon dried rosemary or 1 tablespoon chopped fresh leaves

1 teaspoon dried sage or 1 tablespoon chopped fresh leaves

4 cups boiling water

Honey, for serving (optional)

Lemon slice, for serving (optional)

1. Put the oregano, thyme, rosemary, and sage in a teapot, then cover with the boiling water. Cover with a lid, and steep for 20 minutes.

2. Pour the tisane through a tea strainer into a clean 32-ounce mason jar.

3. Stir in a dash of honey and add a slice of lemon, if desired. Enjoy straight from the jar, or pour into a mug to enjoy. Store any remaining tisane in a covered jar in the refrigerator for up to 4 days.

NOTE: These herbs are easy to find in most grocery stores but are also easy to grow in pots and gardens.

Anti-Inflammatory Green Tea with Ginger

MAKES: 2 cups

Herbalists have hailed the health benefits of green tea for centuries. All true teas are brewed from the dried leaves of the *Camellia sinensis* plant, but green tea is made from unoxidized leaves and is one of the least processed types of tea, helping lock in its medical benefits. It has been shown to provide anti-inflammatory benefits against a variety of diseases, including cancer and diabetes. This recipe pairs it with ginger, which offers a sweet peppery kick and brings further anti-inflammatory benefit.

2 teaspoons green tea

1 teaspoon ginger granules

2 cups boiling water

1. Put the green tea and ginger in a teapot, then cover with the boiling water. Cover with a lid, and steep for 20 minutes.

2. Pour the tea through a tea strainer into a mug and enjoy.

NOTE: This recipe uses dried ginger granules for ease in the infusion technique. Fresh or dried ginger needs to be simmered for 10 minutes before adding to the green tea to steep. Granules can simply steep with the green tea without the extra step of simmering.

Iced Green Tea with Tulsi and Linden

MAKES: 4 cups

This tea combines three herbs that are antioxidant and anti-inflammatory to create a sweet and floral iced tea. Tulsi, also known as holy basil, is a basil plant with sweet floral aroma and taste. It is grounding, centering, and calming without being sedating. It is an adaptogen and antioxidant. Linden blossoms are highly anti-inflammatory, soothing inflamed tissues throughout the body and calming and centering the mind. Linden and tulsi offer complementary flavors to green tea's astringent and slightly bitter nature.

2 teaspoons green tea

2 teaspoons dried linden blossoms

2 teaspoons dried tulsi leaves and flowers

4 cups boiling water

Ice, for serving

Honey, for serving (optional)

1. Put the green tea, linden blossoms, and tulsi in a teapot, then cover with the boiling water. Cover with a lid, and steep for 20 minutes.

2. Pour the tea through a tea strainer into a clean 32-ounce mason jar. Let cool to room temperature.

3. Pour the tea into a glass over ice. Stir in honey to taste, if desired. Store any remaining tea in a covered jar in the refrigerator for up to 4 days.

NOTE: Add a teaspoon of antioxidant and anti-inflammatory hibiscus flowers, dried, to the mix for added cooling effects, tangy flavor, and red color. Another fun way to incorporate hibiscus is in the ice cubes themselves. To do this, make a hibiscus tisane by steeping 1 teaspoon of herb per cup of boiling water, bring to room temperature, strain, and freeze into ice cube trays. Then use these ice cubes to cool this or any other iced tisane.

Milk Thistle Liver-Resilience Tincture

MAKES: 2 cups

Milk thistle seeds have wonderful liver-protecting properties. Their medicinal components do not extract into water, so it is best to make an alcohol-based tincture with them. Even though alcohol is used in the tincture, it is not consumed at a high enough dose to challenge the liver. Any thistle seed can be used interchangeably with milk thistle seed, but milk thistle seeds are relatively large and easy to harvest.

1 cup milk thistle seeds   **2 cups 100-proof vodka**

1. Put the milk thistle seeds in a clean 16-ounce mason jar, then fill the jar with the vodka. Cover with a tight lid, label and let infuse for 6 weeks away from direct sunlight.

2. Line the mouth of a ceramic drip coffee filter with a straining cloth. Pour the tincture through the filter into a clean 2-cup measuring cup with a spout.

3. Pour the tincture through a small funnel into 2 clean (8-ounce) Boston round amber bottles. Cover with tight lids and label. Take a teaspoonful before you expect to expose your liver to undesirable chemicals, large amounts of alcohol, or other things that challenge the health of the liver. Tinctures keep indefinitely due to their alcohol content.

NOTE: Milk thistle tincture is especially helpful for the liver if taken before drinking alcohol, helping process it. To turn this into a pre-party beverage, combine the tincture with 1 cup of bubbly water, the juice of a lime wedge, and 1 cup of lemonade. Stir well, and pour into a glass over ice.

Triple Herb Decoction for Liver and Lymphatic Health

MAKES: 4 cups

The liver and the lymphatic system are hugely important in the body's overall health and resilience, allowing it to eliminate unwanted chemicals in a timely fashion. This decoction contains a trio of herbs that support the body's ability to do so efficiently and effectively.

¼ cup dried burdock root

¼ cup dried red clover blossoms

¼ teaspoon dried licorice root, or more to taste

5 cups water

1. In a saucepot, combine the burdock root, red clover blossoms, licorice root, and water. Bring to a boil.

2. Reduce the heat to a simmer. Simmer for about 40 minutes, or until the liquid has reduced to about 4 cups. Remove from the heat. Cover the pot with a lid, and steep for 20 minutes.

3. Pour the decoction through a tea strainer into a clean 32-ounce mason jar. Enjoy straight from the jar, or pour into a mug to drink. Store any remaining decoction in a covered jar in the refrigerator for up to 4 days.

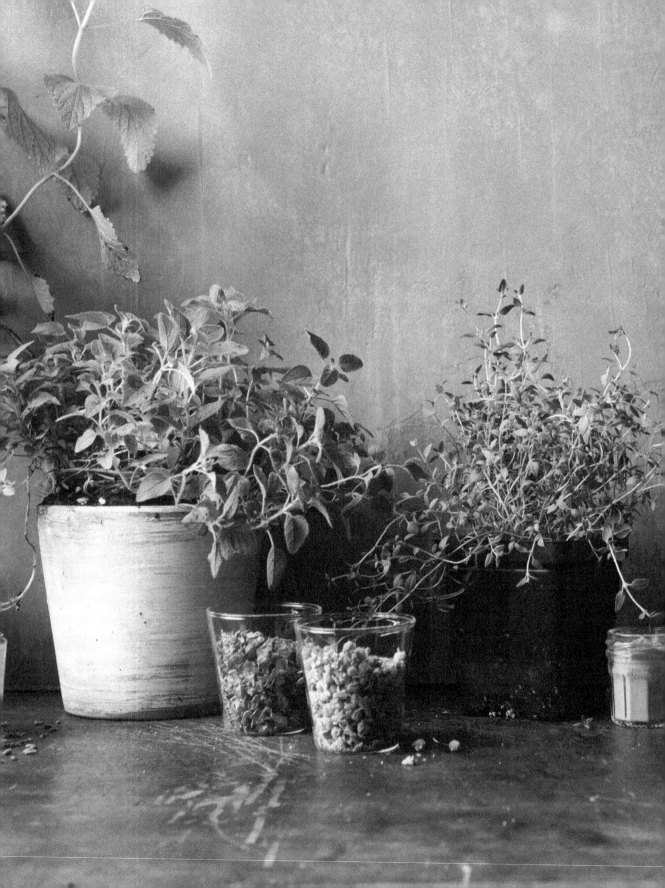

Glossary

Adaptogen: Increases the body's ability to resist the damaging effects of stress and promote or restore normal physiological functioning

Alterative: Favorably alters the course of an ailment, often by supporting the functions of the liver, digestive system, lymph system, and/or kidneys

Analgesic: Producing diminished sensation to pain without loss of consciousness; an herb that is used to relieve pain

Anodyne: Alleviates pain

Antibacterial: Prevents or destroys bacteria, or slows its multiplication

Anticoagulant: Hinders the clotting of blood

Antihistamine: Counteracts histamine in the body; used for treating allergic reactions and cold symptoms

Anti-inflammatory: Reduces the body's immune response to injury, infection, or irritant

Antimutagenic: Reduces the rate of cell mutation, as in cancer cells

Antioxidant: Inhibits oxidation or reactions promoted by oxygen, peroxides, or free radicals

Antispasmodic: Reduces cramping, muscle spasms, and spasmodic pains

Anxiolytic: Relieves anxiety

Astringent: Causes a tightening and toning of soft organic tissues

Bitter: A tincture used to aid digestion, promote the breakdown of foods, and assist in nutrient absorption

Carminative: Expels gas from the stomach or intestines so as to relieve flatulence or abdominal pain or distension

Decoction: A preparation made by boiling the parts of a plant, like bark, roots, stems, and other woody components, in water

Demulcent: Has mucilaginous qualities that are soothing to irritated or inflamed internal tissues

Diaphoretic: Increases perspiration, thereby reducing heat in the body

Diffusive: Tending to break up and distribute

Discutient: Diffusive, especially in cases of cysts and fatty growths

Diuretic: Increases the excretion of urine

Elixir: A sweetened tincture

Emmenagogue: Stimulates menstrual bleeding

Emollient: Making soft or supple

Expectorant: Promotes the discharge or expulsion of mucus from the respiratory tract

Febrifuge: An agent that reduces fever

Galactagogue: Promotes the secretion of breast milk and lactation

Homeostasis: A state of harmonic movement between the different but interdependent groups of elements of the body

Hypoglycemic: Decreases sugar in the blood

Hypotensive: A lowering of blood pressure when it promotes health

Infusion: A type of noncaffeinated herbal tea made by pouring boiling water over delicate parts of the plant, like fruits, leaves, dried flowers, or berries; requires a short steeping time

Lymphagogue: An agent that promotes lymph production and/or lymph flow

Menstruum: Solvent (such as alcohol or vinegar) in which herbs release their properties

Mucilage: The thick, sticky substance inside plants

Nervine: Supporting the health of the entire nervous system; nervous system tonic

Nutritive: Nourishes and builds bodily tissues

Oxymel: A preparation made with a combination of herbs, apple cider vinegar, and honey

Sialagogue: Promotes saliva flow

Tincture: A concentrated herbal preparation made by soaking plant material in alcohol to extract its medicinal benefits

Tisane: A noncaffeinated herbal tea made by pouring boiling water over the plant material to extract its medicinal benefit; requires a longer steeping time than an infusion

Tonic: Increases body tone or tone of specific organs or body systems; invigorates, restores, and refreshes

Vasodilator: Induces or initiates dilation of the blood vessels, improving the ease of blood flow

Vulnerary: Useful in healing wounds

Resources

Herb Distributors

Here are some companies where you can reliably source dried herbs for the recipes in this book. Their products can be ordered direct or found in your local herb shop, or most of them are available via Amazon.

- Frontier Co-op: FrontierCoop.com

- Mountain Rose Herbs: MountainRoseHerbs.com

- Pacific Botanicals: PacificBotanicals.com

- Starwest Botanicals: Starwest-Botanicals.com

Books

Here is a selection of reference books to expand your herbal understanding.

- *Abundantly Well: The Complementary Integrated Medicine Revolution* by Susun S. Weed, 2019.

- *Herbal Medicine for Beginners: Your Guide to Healing Common Ailments with 35 Medicinal Herbs* by Katja Swift and Ryn Midura, 2018.

- *The Herbal Kitchen: Bringing Lasting Health to You and Your Family with 50 Easy-To-Find Common Herbs and Over 250 Recipes* by Kami McBride, 2021.

- *The Herbal Medicine-Maker's Handbook: A Home Manual* by James Green, 2000.

- *The Gift of Healing Herbs: Plant Medicines and Home Remedies for a Vibrantly Healthy Life* by Robin Rose Bennett, 2014.

- *Wild Remedies: How to Forage Healing Foods and Craft Your Own Herbal Medicine* by Rosalee de la Forêt and Emily Han, 2020.

Podcasts

Here is a selection of my favorite herbalism podcasts, including mine! They are full of educational and inspiring information for both home and professional herbalists, and include a variety of interviews with herbalists.

- *Ask Herbal Health Expert Susun Weed* with Susun S. Weed

- *HerbRally* with Mason Hutchison

- *Herbal Radio*, with lectures curated by Mountain Rose Herbs

- *Herbs with Rosalee* with Rosalee de la Forêt

- *The Healthy Herb Podcast* with Brighid Doherty

- *The Holistic Herbalism Podcast* with Katja Swift and Ryn Midura

References

Bond, Timothy J., and Emma J. Derbyshire "Rooibos Tea and Health: A Systematic Review of the Evidence from the Last Two Decades." *Nutrition and Food Technology* 6, no. 1 (June 2020): 1–11. sciforschenonline.org/journals /nutrition-food/article-data/NFTOA166/NFTOA166.pdf.

Brinker, Frances. *Herbal Contraindications and Drug Interactions plus Herbal Adjuncts with Medicines.* Sandy, OR: Eclectic Medical Publications, 2010.

Carabotti, Marilia, Annunziata Scirocco, Maria Antoinetta Maselli, and Carola Severi. "The Gut-Brain Axis: Interactions between Enteric Microbiota, Central and Enteric Nervous Systems." *Annals of Gastroenterology* 28, no. 2 (April–June 2015): 203–9. ncbi.nlm.nih.gov/pmc/articles/PMC4367209.

Cox, Tracy. "Higher Mushroom Consumption Is Associated with a Lower Risk of Cancer." Penn State University. April 21, 2021. PSU.edu/news/research /story/higher-mushroom-consumption-associated-lower-risk-cancer.

Dietz, Christina, and Matthijs Dekker. "Effect of Green Tea Phytochemicals on Mood and Cognition." *Current Pharmaceutical Design* 23, no. 19 (2017): 2876–2905. doi.org/10.2174/1381612823666170105151800.

Galeotti, Nicoletta, Elisa Vivoli, Anna Rita Bilia, Franco Francesco Vincieri, and Carla Ghelardini. "St. John's Wort Reduces Neuropathic Pain through a Hypericin-Mediated Inhibition of the Protein Kinase Cgamma and Epsilon Activity." *Biochemical Pharmacology* 79, no. 9 (May 2010): 1327–36. doi.org/10.1016/j.bcp.2009.12.016.

Galleano, Monica, Patricia I. Oteiza, and Cesar G. Fraga. "Cocoa, Chocolate and Cardiovascular Disease." *Journal of Cardiovascular Pharmacology* 54, no. 6 (December 2009): 483–90. doi.org/10.1097/FJC.0b013e3181b76787.

Gardner, Zoe, and Michael McGuffin, eds. *American Herbal Products Association's Botanical Safety Handbook.* 2nd ed. Silver Spring, MD: CRC Press, 2013.

Jalalyazdi, Majid, Javad Ramezani, Azadeh Izadi-Moud, Fereshteh Madani-Sani, Shokufeh Shahlaei, and Shirin Sadat Ghiasi. "Effect of *Hibiscus sabdariffa* on Blood Pressure in Patients with Stage 1 Hypertension." *Journal of Advanced*

Pharmaceutical Technology & Research 10, no. 3 (July–September 2019): 107–11. doi.org/10.4103/japtr.JAPTR_402_18.

Kennedy, David O., Bernd Bonnländer, Stefanie C. Lang, Ivo Pischel, Joanne Forster, Julie Khan, Philippa A. Jackson, and Emma L. Wightman. "Acute and Chronic Effects of Green Oat (*Avena sativa*) Extract on Cognitive Function and Mood during a Laboratory Stressor in Healthy Adults: A Randomised, Double-Blind, Placebo-Controlled Study in Healthy Humans." *Nutrients* 12, no. 6 (June 2020): 1598. doi.org/10.3390/nu12061598.

Kuo, Jip, Kenny Wen-Chyuan Chen, I-Shiung Cheng, Pu-Hsi Tsai, Ying-Jui Lu, and Ning-Yuean Lee. "The Effect of Eight Weeks of Supplementation with *Eleutherococcus senticosus* on Endurance Capacity and Metabolism in Human." *The Chinese Journal of Physiology* 53, no. 2 (April 2010): 105–11. doi.org/10.4077/cjp.2010.amk018.

Qin, Qiaojing, Jianying Niu, Zhaoxia Wang, Wangjie Xu, Zhongdong Qiao, and Yong Gu. "*Astragalus membranaceus* Extract Activates Immune Response in Macrophages via Heparanase." *Molecules* 17, no. 6 (June 2012): 7232–40. doi.org/10.3390/molecules17067232.

Silberstein, R. B., A. Pipingas, J. Song, D. A. Camfield, P. J. Nathan, and C. Stough. "Examining Brain-Cognition Effects of *Gingko biloba* Extract: Brain Activation in the Left Temporal and Left Prefrontal Cortex in an Object Working Memory Task." *Evidence-Based Complementary and Alternative Medicine* (2011): 164139. doi.org/10.1155/2011/164139.

Walker, Ann F., Georgios Marakis, Andrew P. Morris, and Paul A. Robinson. "Promising Hypotensive Effect of Hawthorn Extract: A Randomized Double-Blind Pilot Study of Mild, Essential Hypertension." *Phytotherapy Research* 16, no. 1 (February 2002): 48–54. doi.org/10.1002/ptr.947.

Zakay-Rones, Z., E. Thom, T. Wollan, and J. Wadstein. "Randomized Study of the Efficacy and Safety of Oral Elderberry Extract in the Treatment of Influenza A and B Virus Infections." *The Journal of International Medical Research* 32, no. 2 (March–April 2004): 132–40. doi.org/10.1177/147323000403200205.

Index

Acknowledgments

Thank you, Adrian Potts, Meredith Tennant, and the others at Callisto Media for helping me create this book.

Thank you, Susun Weed, my mentor, for introducing me to the Wise Woman Tradition of Healing and new ways to understand health, wholeness, and holiness. Thank you, Katja Swift, my business mentor, for inspiring me to attain my goals and dreams.

To Bernard, my love, and Isla Rose, my dear daughter, thank you for your support and for allowing me time to devote to this project.

Thank you to the plants for gifts of health, beauty, and lessons on how to be in relationship with Earth and her beings with humility and grace.

About the Author

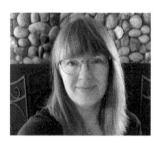 Brighid Doherty is a community herbalist and the founder of the Solidago School of Herbalism. For more than two decades, she has worked with plants in a variety of ways: as a student, teacher, gardener-forager, medicine maker, and health consultant. She offers information and inspiration to home herbalists through workshops, medicinal plant walks, and *The Healthy Herb Podcast*. Brighid's online course, Nourish Yourself, teaches people how to infuse common herbs into daily life in simple ways with nourishing herbal infusions. An herbalist who works within the Wise Woman Tradition of Healing, she empowers others to be more self-reliant in their health and healing. For more information, you can visit her website, SolidagoHerbSchool.com, and follow her on Instagram @solidagoherbschool.

CPSIA information can be obtained
at www.ICGtesting.com
Printed in the USA
JSHW060454190922
30616JS00001B/1

9 781638 784807